The Art of
Growing
a Beard

The Art of Growing a Beard

by
Marvin Grosswirth

Illustrations by Albert Siringo

HARPER & ROW, PUBLISHERS
New York, Evanston, San Francisco, London

A hardcover edition of this book is published by Jarrow Press, Inc. It is here reprinted by arrangement.

First BARNES & NOBLE BOOKS edition published 1975.

STANDARD BOOK NUMBER: 06–465046–4

75 10 9 8 7 6 5 4 3 2 1

To Howard, who will find this
book useful all too soon.

ACKNOWLEDGMENTS

Among those responsible for the realization of this book are:

Philip Deemer, who originated the idea; Arthur J. Goldsmith, Jr., who supported it; Mrs. Marianne S. Andersen, who is apparently making a career of editing male-oriented books; John Gangi, editor of *Men's Hairstylist & Barber's Journal,* and J. Nelson Snyder, Secretary of the Associated Master Barbers and Beauticians of America, both of whom contributed to the research; the incredible staff of the Mid-Manhattan Branch of the New York Public Library, for whom no question is too outlandish or obscure; and, most important, my wife, Marilyn: chief assistant researcher, copy editor, proofreader, idea tester, tantrum cooler, shock absorber, firm taskmaster, and gentle critic.

New York, June 1971   M.G.

TABLE OF CONTENTS

FOREWORD   13
     by Commander Edward Whitehead
INTRODUCTION   20
1. A CLIPPED HISTORY OF THE BEARD   25
2. THE BEARD IN LANGUAGE, LORE,   34
   AND LEGEND
     In the Beginning Was the Word
     Historical Oddities
     Religious Beards
     Artistic Beards
     Some Other Famous Beards
     The Superlative Beard
3. A GLOSSARY OF THE BEARD   48
     Hippie-Freakie; Rabbinical/Eastern
     Orthodox; Full Beard; Partial-Full
     Beard; Pennsylvania Dutch; Lincoln-
     esque; Ring-Frame; Vandyke; Goatee;
     Oriental Scholar; Underlip; Mephisto-
     phelian; Ring Beard
     Miscellaneous Topiary
4. HAIRY ANCILLARIES   64
     RAF; Handlebar; Soup-Strainer; Balkan;
     Stalinesque; Brush; Lip Rester; Latin;
     Miscellaneous
     Some Notes about Sideburns
     Making the Connection

5. SELECTING A BEARD 73
6. PLOTTING THE BEARD 81
    Preparation
    Outlining
    Shaving
7. THE GESTATION PERIOD 90
    A Beard of a Different Color
    Itching
    Coping with Objections
    Children
8. CARE AND FEEDING OF THE BEARD 99
    Washing
    Combing and Brushing
    Trimming
    Gouges, Holes, and Bald Spots
    Trimming the Mustache
    Cosmetics, Lotions, and Potions
    Cleaning Up
    Professional Care
9. THE SENSUOUS BEARD 112
    Your Beard and Your Woman
    The Beard on the Prowl
    Bearded Lovemaking
    Kissing
10. THE ART OF WEARING A BEARD 120
    The Beard as a Hobby
    The Beard as a Symbol of Strength
    The Beard as a Life-Style

The Art of
Growing
a Beard

FOREWORD

From time to time, over the past 20 years, I have been invited to write a definitive book on beards. Largely because I have been preoccupied in other directions I have not accepted the challenge, and I have put it aside with the vague idea of tackling it in my dotage.

Meanwhile, I am glad to contribute this Foreword to Marvin Grosswirth's scholarly work on the same subject.

I became acquainted with the author when he, in his role of chairman of New York's MENSA, invited me to address that organization on a subject of my own choosing. I took advantage of the occasion to test the validity of a thesis on which I was in the process of writing a book. *The Human Factor — How To Succeed By Really Trying* is a subject on which I have frequently spoken; now that I was expanding the text of the speech into a book, it was obviously valuable for me to bounce my ideas off the minds of a group of people in the top 2% of the national I.Q. range.

Though my forthcoming book has little to say on beards, there is some overlap of subject matter. For instance, I refer briefly to beards in a chapter on *Style*, or, to use an older word that I prefer, "panache." I consider style, or panache, an important attribute of the successful man in any field. (I define "success" not as self-aggrandizement, or the acquisition of wealth and power, but as self-development and, ultimately, self-fulfillment.)

The original medieval meaning of the word panache was "a tuft or plume of feathers worn in the helmet." It is not overstretching the point to translate that, in contemporary terms, as a tuft of hair worn on the chin. Thus, a beard is very much in line with present-day manifestations of style or panache. The author touches upon this point, and I should like to give it additional emphasis; especially as most men inclined to follow the advice offered in this book are probably also seeking to make a success of their lives.

This aspect of the subject is, to me, an indelible part of the case for growing a beard, and it has parallel bearing on the subject of conformity. In this day and age, when beards are still in the minority, nonconformity is a corollary of the case for beards.

I am an enthusiastic advocate of independence of mind, of individual initiative, of the wisdom of taking a line of one's own. Successful men in all walks of life tend to possess not only a strong character, but a high degree of individuality as well. Few are colorless conformists. Some are allowed mild idiosyncrasies, others are acknowledged eccentrics, a few are out-and-out cranks.

14

This is even truer in Britain, where we tolerate, if not encourage, the eccentric rather more freely. But in England the word "crank" means something a little different from the crotchety, irascible type usually so designated in this country. According to George Bernard Shaw, a crank was any man who had made up his mind on any subject whatsoever. But he was hypercritical.

Please don't imagine that I advocate eccentricity as an end in itself. Oddity for its own sake, with nothing to support it, has nothing to commend it. But I do advocate taking a line of one's own in one sphere, *provided* it is indicative of a similar capacity in other areas. I stress the need to act independently, to question the majority view, to maintain one's critical faculty, to make decisions based on one's own findings and to follow through.

This independence of mind can be manifested in many ways; growing a beard is just one of them. And it is important to remember that an attitude of mind is best expressed in action. Appearances, per se, do not mean much. I am against the growing of beards by every Tom, Dick and Harry.

Many years ago Mitch Miller told me, when a few of us, all bearded, were gathered together to discuss the subject on his radio program, that he had grown his beard when he had played the oboe in an orchestra. His friends had ridiculed his efforts to express himself in this way and he would have shaved it off, but for his wife, who said, "You are a very good oboe player; you should keep it."

15

This provided me with a first-class illustration of my argument against indiscriminate beard growing. A man must have at least *begun* to assert himself, to prove his mettle, before he lays down the gauntlet quite so obtrusively.

Subject to this caveat, I can muster arguments for whiskers that I didn't dream existed when, in September, 1939 (a good year for beards), I heard that Britain had declared war. Spontaneously I threw my razor over the side, and vowed not to shave again until victory was ours. During the ensuing six years my beard served to keep the cold out in northern latitudes and the mosquitoes at bay in the South Pacific.

When, eventually, I left the Royal Navy, I retained my beard because I'd become attached to it—or it to me. My wife, who liked it, and my children, who grew up swinging on it, wouldn't hear of my shaving it off; and I, not caring much what other people thought, hung on to it.

During the postwar years in England beards were not especially common, but no one saw fit to question my right to retain mine. It was not, so to speak, a conversation piece. In fact, it was not until I arrived in New York in January, 1953, that my whiskers came into their own. During my first few weeks in New York I was mistaken, variously, for Thor Heyerdahl, the Deity, and others well known for hirsute adornment. But, once I had been persuaded to participate in my own advertising, there was no further occasion for mistaken identity.

Thereafter I found myself being interviewed and haranguing audiences on a wide variety of subjects. Invariably, however, the subject of beards would crop up and I would be closely — but always politely — questioned on the subject.

Finding myself cast in the role of judge at occasional beard-growing competitions, usually on TV, my prejudice against indiscriminate beard growing slowly hardened. It became all too apparent that some men can't grow a beard, and should not be encouraged to try. I am now firmly of the opinion that this male equivalent of a woman's crowning glory (the only thing left that a man can do and a woman can't) should be reserved for men with at least a semblance of fire in their blood, men with intestinal fortitude, men who feel a compulsion to right wrongs, *men who are prepared to back up their challenge.*

In those days, as now (to a lesser extent), the conforming beard was obsolete. Only the defiant beard existed — the beard against the wind. This element of defiance, or sublime self-assurance, lurks behind every beard, and that is as it should be. The beard and the challenge are inseparable.

I cannot do better than quote, from memory, George Bernard Shaw's reply to a letter from the manufacturers of a well-known electric razor. They had written to him stating that they had heard rumors to the effect that he was proposing to remove his beard. They would be highly flattered to think that the Shaw chin was to be shaved by one of their razors, they said, and were sending him their latest model.

Shaw's reply, on a postcard—he never wrote more unless he was paid for it—was along these lines:

"I am returning your razor, as I have no intention of using it, or of removing my beard. I am keeping it for the reason that I grew it. I grew it for the same reason that my father grew his. I have a clear recollection of asking him that question, and of his reply. I was about five at the time, and I was standing at my father's knee whilst he was shaving. I said to him, 'Daddy, why do you shave?' He looked at me in silence for a full minute, before throwing his razor out the window, saying, 'Why the hell do I?' He never did again."

Since my arrival in New York nearly 20 years ago, hair styles of the American male have undergone vast changes. *Life* magazine, in an editorial on the subject a few years ago, attributed this to the Beatles and to me. Whether or not they were justified in laying this metamorphosis at the door of the British, they were certainly right in saying that beards had spread across America like crabgrass across a lawn in summer.

This, you will have gathered, is not in line with my aims and beliefs. But if you, dear reader, can categorize yourself as an achiever, one who is going to cut a swathe and carve out a niche for himself, go to it.

May your shadow never grow less.

Commander Edward Whitehead, C. B. E.

He that hath a beard is more than a youth,
  and he that hath no beard is less than a man.

— Much Ado About Nothing,
            ACT THREE, SCENE II

The glory of a face is its beard.

                — The Talmud

INTRODUCTION

One evening not long ago, while I was engrossed in my nocturnal ablutions, I felt a mounting sense of annoyance with my beard, which for some inexplicable reason refused to allow itself to be evenly trimmed. Finally, in a fit of pique, I savagely applied shears and blade, and a few seconds later I was smooth-jawed. (Mercifully, some divine intervention stayed my hand when it came to the mustache.) My wife, who was at the time a bride of less than one year, refused to allow me to come to bed. Ultimately, her innate sense of compassion prevailed, and she relented.

One could hardly blame her. Ordinary prudence dictates that any attractive young woman of good sense will avoid sleeping with a man who is, for all practical purposes, a total stranger. And stranger I was. For one thing, I looked quite different: my wife had never seen me beardless. For another, intermixed with the luxuriant tufts of hair clogging the drain were sizable chunks of my personality. The pain was indescribable. I had not realized how very much a part of me my beard had become and I yearned for some immediate means of restoring it to its original state, a condition which, through great patience, I was ultimately able to accomplish. I vowed never again to remove my beard unless compelled to do so by some unknown and as yet unimaginable calamity.

Nor was the pain entirely psychological. I had forgotten how much it hurts to drag a strip of honed metal across one's face. I used to jest that it took me eight minutes to shave: three for the removal of stubble and another five to stanch the flow of blood. To my dismay, the bad joke came back to haunt me with agonizing reality.

My beard is about seven years old, its birth roughly coinciding with the demise of my first marriage. There is considerable significance in pairing the two events, as you shall soon see.

Shortly after I reembarked on the turbulent sea of bachelorhood, I decided to succumb to the urge which, at one time or another, obsesses all men: the desire to grow facial adornment. I had already cultivated a mustache of which any hussar or Balkan field marshal could be proud, but growing a beard was quite another matter. I realized that for at least a short period of time I would be something of a social pariah (see Chapter 7), not an easy circumstance to be confronted by a newly made bachelor *in extremis*. After some six months of success—ranging from moderate to poor—with the opposite sex, I was on the verge of breaking what tenuous ties existed by appearing in public with a stubbly chin, a characteristic unfairly but unfailingly associated with the less desirable elements of society. It required a certain amount of courage on my part — as it will require on yours — but I made the happy discovery that it was well worth it, and I have no doubt that you will make that same discovery.

My beard took approximately three weeks before it began to look like a beard ought. Rapidly and perceptibly, my social life underwent a significant change. Where I had managed previously to establish contact with rather insipid, somewhat vapid, husband-hunting girls, I now found myself locked in conversation and other activities with *women* — sophisticated, worldly women who had Experienced Life, had Been Around; women who demanded of their men intelligence, wit, passion and compassion, and little else. Not one of them ever accused me of being "handsome" or "attractive." But almost all of them have at one time or another described me as looking "interesting." To be considered interesting by a woman is to be given a key which unlocks myriad doors. (See Chapter 9.)

Women are not the only ones who find my face interesting. I have been asked to pose for painters, photographers, and sculptors — all total strangers — who have approached me at parties, on the street, in museums, and in concert halls. Not one has ever treated me with anything less than respect and deference. I shall always cherish the memory of the slightly dowdy, heavily accented matron who approached me one afternoon in the Museum of Modern Art in New York and asked, obviously awestruck: "Are you *some*body?" I informed her that indeed I was and walked on, leaving her to ponder exactly who I might be.

Not all the benefits of being bearded are social. At about the time I assumed anew the burdens of bachelorhood, I also took on a new career. I obtained employment with a small but ambitious publishing firm (not the publishers of the present work) engaged in the production, for other publishers, of religious books. I gave two weeks' notice to my old employer and promptly stored away my razor, so that by the time I was ready to begin the new job, my beard was already moderately presentable. It proved to be a great asset. Most of the people with whom I came into contact professionally seemed to feel that my beard lent an aura of sincerity and authenticity to my sales promotion efforts. Some even assumed that I was a professional religionist or, at the very least, a scholar. I did nothing to perpetuate such mistaken assumptions and even tried to correct them when they were brought out into the open; but I found that people want to believe what they want to believe, and only a gross, graceless man would disabuse them of an article of faith without very good cause. The wisdom of this attitude was demonstrated to me not long ago in front of the Israel Museum in Jerusalem.

A well-meaning museum guard whose intentions were the best but whose English was not, had attempted to explain some aspect of Hebraic folklore to a church group from the American Midwest. Later, on the steps, when I saw the group emerging, I took it upon myself to clear away some of the confusion which the guard had engendered. When I had finished, I was thanked profusely and asked what university I was connected with. After assuring the good people that I was not a scholar and was in Israel on business, I left, but not before overhearing the leader of the group explain to his flock: "He says he's not with a school. Must be connected with the Museum." I decided, for social as well as ecumenical reasons, to allow the myth to stand.

Even in moments of solitude, my beard has been a comfort to me. It is warm and soft and enjoys being stroked or gently scratched. As a hobby, a beard is far more rewarding than, say, stamp collecting, because it is alive, vital, dynamic, and constantly changing. Within the same basic contours, I can change my beard every two or three weeks, wearing it long or short, full or sparse, mustache connected or detached, sideburns ditto; in short, when mental blocks or physical lassitude prevent my expressing my creativity on paper, I can always resort to my chin. (See Chapter 10.)

And so can you. The right beard, worn well, is a mark of virility, distinction, dash, and self-confidence. Does any man, especially *you*, deserve less?

1. A CLIPPED HISTORY OF THE BEARD

From the very beginning, the beard has always figured significantly in the history of Western civilization. Artistic representations of the Lord God Jehovah, who created man in His own image, always show Him with a beard. The earliest authenticated records, however, are of the ancient Egyptians, who grew beards and lovingly curled, braided, and dyed them. Even when actual chin growth fell from fashion, Egyptian monarchs, male and female alike, wore the *postiche*, a false beard made of gold or other metal and fastened to a gold chin strap, which was in turn attached to a ribbon tied about the

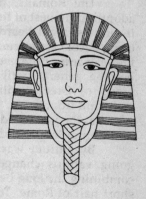

head. This style was popular from about 3000 B.C. to about 1580 B.C.

The ancient Mesopotamian civilizations lavished much attention on their beards. The Persians and Assyrians resorted to dyes and they, as well as the Chaldeans, Babylonians, and Medians, devoted many hours to oiling, curling, plaiting, and decorating their beards, often with gold thread and dust. Perfumes and starches were especially popular during festivals. In ancient India and Turkey, the beard was an emblem of position and sagacity. Only boors and slaves shaved, and to pull a man's beard was to court death.

The curled, luxuriant beards of ancient Greece flourished until 323 B.C., when Alexander the Great decreed that his soldiers shave them off, lest they provide ready handles for the enemy. It was a time, obviously, when combat was somewhat more intimate than it is today.

The Romans, true to their tradition of adopting the best of the Greeks and romanizing it, grew straight beards, regarding the Hellenic chin decor as effeminate. According to the *Encyclopaedia Britannica*, ". . . shaving did not become general until about 454 B.C., when a group of Greek Sicilian barbers came to the mainland from Sicily." This would seem to indicate that the venerated Italian barber is indeed a tradition of long standing.

Byzantium was no less bearded, undergoing various changes in style, but basically combining the long beard of the Orient with the short hair of Rome. Toward the end of the 12th century, however, influence had shifted to Florence and Venice, which became the fashion centers for the rest of Europe.

Beards were also popular among the Anglo-Saxons, but with the coming of Christianity in the 7th century, the clergy were ordered to go abroad clean-shaven. William the Conqueror, the first Norman king of England (1066-87), compelled his courtiers to remove their traditional mustaches and, in keeping with the Norman style, remained facially unadorned until the Crusades, when the knights, like soldiers everywhere, apparently felt no need to maintain the amenities of fashion in the field. They were, perhaps, also influenced by the styles of the vanquished Orientals who placed great store by their beards. To this day, the beard carries great distinction among Muslims.

For the next five hundred years, the European beard led a tenuous, on-again, off-again existence. Styles varied greatly, ranging from the face-framing fringe of Henry VIII to the miniscule *mouche*, the little tuft of lip hair affected by the French and Dutch cavaliers. From this chaos, a kind of order finally emerged. Louis XIII, King of France (1610-1643), began losing his hair and popularized the powdered wig. It was apparently too

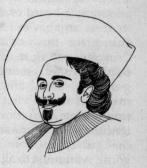

complicated to attend to these ornate head-dresses and worry about beards and mustaches as well, and facial hair became virtually unknown for nearly two hundred years.

Eventually, the powdered wig made its way across the turbulent Atlantic and found a home in the American Colonies. The Spanish *conquistadores*, the great Dutch and English explorers, John Cabot, Samuel Champlain, Captain John Smith — all of them were endowed with rich chin growths. But by the time the Colonies were ready to declare their independence, the powdered wig and the bare chin had taken firm hold. None of the signers of the Declaration of Independence or of the Constitution wore a smidgen of hair on their faces. (Edward Rutledge of South Carolina is sometimes cited as an exception. Mr. Rutledge affected a hair style in which he combed his rather long tresses over his forehead and cheeks so that they could be seen in front of his ears. Strictly speaking, however, this cannot be regarded as a beard or mustache; his lip and chin were clean-shaven.) So unusual were beards during the Birth of the Nation that Elizabeth Drinker, writing in 1794 about a visit to Philadelphia, listed among the curiosities she had seen an elephant and two bearded men on the streets. A recent visit to that city by the author would seem to indicate that, except for the absence of the elephant, the situation has not changed appreciably.

As it must to all extreme modes of fashion, disfavor came to the powdered wig. Born in France, it died there as well when the revolutionary National Assembly prohibited styles of dress designed to underline social differences. Short hair became the fashion and quickly traversed the ocean. The beard, however, did not return until about half a century later.

Authorities are uncertain as to what precipitated facial growth as a fashion. Victorian London established the pattern around 1840, but it took some 15 years for the style to take hold in the United States. Uncle Sam, symbol of America, did not sprout whiskers until 1858, and Abraham Lincoln, the first president to wear a beard, grew his between his nomination for the post and his inauguration. A wide variety of beards and mustaches flourished during the Lincoln era, particularly during the Civil War. One innovator not only contributed to American history; he gave his name, in a somewhat convoluted state, to the language. In 1843, a young cadet, Ambrose E. Burnside, entered the U.S. Military Academy at West Point, displaying a lush growth along his cheeks. He eventually rose to the rank of general and became an important figure in the War Between the States. His bushy locks came to be known as "burnsides," which some misguided folk etymologist decided should rightly be called sideburns (because, you see, they are worn on

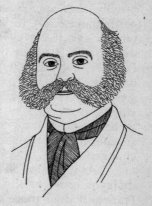

the sides). The word has ever since meant hair growing in front of the ears and along the cheeks.

Everyone wore a beard in the Lincoln era and the years immediately following. No physician would dream of going beardless; soldiers and bankers wore beards; actors and professors sported them; politicians great and small grew whiskers; all men of substance were facially hirsute. So, unfortunately, were some notorious types of ignoble character, such as the quacks who purveyed nostrums and panaceas, all the while wearing beards in an attempt to present a portrait of respectability and reliability.

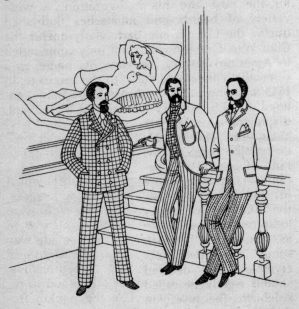

Waiting for the ladies.

The styles were as varied as the wearers: splayed and spaded, split, curled, turned upward, turned downward, full-faced, bare-chinned (exposing a small, round, bald patch surrounded by growth); the thin, pointed, droopy-mustached-type inspired by Napoleon III and sported by the unfortunate General Custer and the popu-lar Buffalo Bill Cody; long sideburns cascading downward to be met by the upward sweep of the lavish mustache, a style dubbed the "Franz Josef" in tribute to the Emperor of Aus-tria; all of these and many more decorated the chins of American men in the years follow-ing the Civil War. Free enterprise was not long in recognizing the trend, inventing needs result-ing from it and then ful-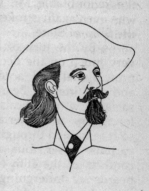filling those needs. There were products which assured the user a full beard in six weeks. Buckingham's Dye and Ayer's Hair Vigor were designed to disguise premature whiteness in beards. Even the rules of etiquette made way for the beard. *Hill's Manual of Social and Business Forms*, published in 1879, admonished readers: "Never allow butter, soup or other food to re-main in your whiskers. Use the napkin fre-quently." Sound advice, despite its age.

31

The surge of *pogonophilia* or *pogonomania* (see next chapter) began to subside with the century. Each president who followed Lincoln was bearded, except for the unfortunate Andrew Johnson. Then, in 1884, Grover Cleveland, heavily mustached but nude of chin, entered the White House. The executive beard had one last gasp in 1888 when Benjamin Harrison was elected; but he was defeated four years later by the redoubtable Mr. Cleveland, and no beard was ever again stroked by a hand that steered the Ship of State.

By the turn of the century, beards were very much on the decline, worn only by a few professional and academic types, the artistic, and the literati. Beards soon came to be associated with radicals, Bolsheviks, Bohemians, foreigners, and other alleged undesirables. And so it remained through two World Wars and the various lesser, but always prevalent, armed conflicts of the 20th century until today, when beards are undergoing a remarkable resurgence.

Readers old enough to grow a beard are doubtlessly acquainted with the most recent history of chin decor, obviating the need to detail it here. To summarize, then: The beatniks of the 50's and 60's seem to have started the trend, later to be picked up by the hippies of the late 60's. Madison Avenue sported neatly trimmed beards for a short time, but there it was more of a fad than a trend. When many of the beatniks and hippies tired of "dropping out" and rejoined the Establishment, they brought with them some of the quaint customs and mores of their erstwhile counterculture, including their facial fringes. At first only acceptable in such esoteric circles as publishing, communications, the arts, and some areas of education, beards became more and more universal; by now it is neither unusual nor surprising to find them in some of the most conservative establishments, such as banking houses, brokerage firms, and insurance companies.

There is, perhaps, another reason for the current proliferation of beards. In very recent years, the male fashion industry has finally managed to achieve its conglomerate heart's desire: the introduction of high style in men's clothes. At this writing, the white shirt, the gray flannel suit, the conservative tie, and the wing-tip shoe are virtual museum pieces. As has happened so often in Western history, man has again allowed his basic peacock instincts to flourish. Does it not seem natural that any man ready—indeed, *anxious*—to decorate his body with manmade fibers should not also want to do so with God-given hair? Thus, many men who have grown beards for the sheer novelty of it, or to be "in," are discovering the multiple benefits and pleasures of a well-covered chin, all of which we shall explore in the following chapters.

2. THE BEARD IN LANGUAGE, LORE, AND LEGEND

In the Beginning Was the Word

Although the English language is heavily infused with a high percentage of Latin, approximately 80% of all *spoken* English derives from the Anglo-Saxon. Thus, the most common words, including those for various parts of the body, are generally more closely related to the Germanic than to the Romance languages. The fancy nomenclature for private parts is all Latin. The earthier, more popular four-letter words are venerable Anglo-Saxon, reaching back in history to Chaucer and beyond. *Beard* is no exception.

Webster's Third International Dictionary gives the origin of *beard* as Middle English *berd* from Old English *beard*—which would seem to indicate some orthographic regression—from Old High German *bart*. Not surprisingly, *Bart* is the modern German word for beard. In French, Spanish, Italian, and Portuguese, the word for beard is a variation of the Latin *barba* (which, however, has nothing to do with *barbarian*).

Predictably, the Greeks, too, had a word for it: *pōgōn*. As prefix, it supplies such esoteric words as *pogonology*, which describes the very book you are now reading. Its author, therefore, is a *pogonologist*. Should you desire to provoke a clean-shaven and less literate friend, simply accuse him publicly of committing *pogonotomy*. If he threatens to become violent, reassure him that the word refers to the act of shaving. He will probably not believe you. It is hoped that when you have finished reading this book, you will undertake the worthwhile and satisfying avocation of *pogonotrophy*, beard-growing.

Using the *pogon-* prefix, it is possible to construct one's own words, all perfectly good English. *Pogonophilia* and *pogonomania*, used in the preceding chapter, are the author's inventions. If your wife or girlfriend offers resistance to your attempts at pogonotrophy, you may rightly claim that she suffers from *pogonophobia*. (If both ladies are *pogonophobes*, you might do well to seek some other attachments, as it is clear that neither of them understands you.)

Mustache, or *moustache*, as it is often spelled, is also Greek in origin. Eric Partridge (*Origins*; New York, 1948: The Macmillan Co.) traces it back to the Greek *mustakhos*, upper lip. The Spanish have immortalized the hirsute adornment of the *mustakhos* with the proverb: "A kiss without a mustache is like an egg without salt."

Whiskers are rather tenuously related to *Verge*, according to Partridge and others. The original Medieval Latin meaning was "a supple branch or twig," but the etymology for the word is too full of "perhapses" and "possiblys" for any genuine conviction about its derivation.

At least three types of whiskers are named for people. A Flemish painter who lived in the first part of the 17th century painted so many aristocrats with small, pointed beards that the style came to be known as the Vandyke, after the artist. General Burnside also added his name to the language, as described in the preceding chapter. A particularly lavish and full style of sideburns was exhibited by Lord Dundreary, a character in *Our American Cousin*, a play best remembered as the one Mr. Lincoln was attending the night John Wilkes Booth did his dastardly deed. The sideburn style lived on, however, and was known as "dundrearys" in America. Englishmen preferred referring to them as "mutton chops" or "Picadilly weepers."

Surprisingly, the only apparent usage of the word *beard* in slang is in connection with female pubic hair, and even that persisted only in the late 17th—early 18th centuries. Thus, a "beard-splitter" was a slang term describing a Don Juan—or his equipment. It is entirely proper that the use of the term "beard" for so feminine an attribute should fall out of favor and into disuse.

36

Historical Oddities

The absence of beards in slang is matched by a similar paucity in mythology and legend, where they are mentioned or depicted only when the particular style of a given time so dictates. Thus, when beards were popular in a culture or period, they appeared significantly in the art of that period. The gods of mythology are either clean-shaven or bearded, depending on what was in vogue when the particular statue or painting was made.

But the dictates of fashion extended far beyond the world of art. When beards were popular in ancient Greece, it was frequently possible to discern a man's occupation or station by the cut of his facial hair. Philosophers wore "long, flowing beards"; historians wore short ones, and the Epicureans emulated the philosophers, with beards to match their long, curly locks. The Stoics simply allowed theirs to grow at will, as it were.

Conformity to style can become oppressive, as many of today's hairy youth can testify. In 1705, Peter the Great decreed that the wearing of beards at court was not to be permitted. Some reluctant courtiers who failed to respond to the ukase with suitable alacrity had their chins shaved with oyster knives, a device not recommended for delicate skin. Ordinary citizens who wished to continue wearing their beards were required to pay a tax. Some Russians, fearful of not being recognized in heaven, preserved their shorn whiskers in boxes and were buried with them. Others preferred leaving Mother Russia to shaving. Peter's daughter-in-law, Catherine the Great, repealed the law in 1765, to much acclaim and celebration, enhancing her already legendary reputation as an admirer of things masculine.

Further evidence of oppression can be found in Leominster, Massachusetts, on the tombstone of one Joseph Palmer. It bears the inscription: "Persecuted for growing the beard." The visage peering from the marker is that of a benign individual with foliage worthy of a modern department store Santa Claus. The un-

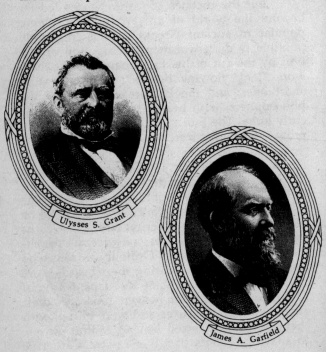

Ulysses S. Grant

James A. Garfield

fortunate Mr. Palmer grew his beard in 1840. Had he but waited 20 years, he would have been at the height of fashion: Abraham Lincoln took office in 1861 with a well-covered chin. In addition to Mr. Lincoln, Ulysses S. Grant (1869-1877), Rutherford B. Hayes (1877-1881), James A. Garfield (1881), and Benjamin Harrison (1889-1893) all eschewed shaving while in the White House. King George V (1910-1936) was the last monarch of the British Empire to wear a beard, and Napoleon III (1852-1870) was the last

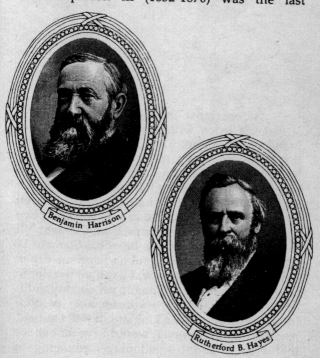

Benjamin Harrison

Rutherford B. Hayes

monarch of France to wear one, which is no great distinction as he was the last monarch of France, period. (Not counting Charles de Gaulle, of course.)

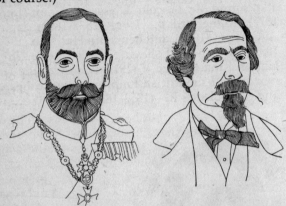

As are most things French, the lore of *la barbe* is laden with intrigue and adventure. Francis I, for example, is credited with initiating the mode for beards in the early 16th century, but there are conflicting stories concerning the origins of his beard. One source claims that Francis was inspired by Julius II, who ascended the papal throne in 1503 and was the first pope to wear a beard. Every pope from Clement VII in 1523 to Clement IX was bearded. Clement IX ended the trend in 1667, and no pope since then has worn a beard. Julius was a valiant warrior in God's cause, and his dynamic personality, military strength, and not inconsiderable political influence were assets a king might well emulate. Another story, however, would have us believe that Francis and his entourage, engaging in some good-natured Yuletide horseplay on the Feast of the Epiphany, 1521, pelted the chateau of his rival, the Comte de Saint-Pol, with snowballs. The Comte's guests retaliated with a fusillade of ripe fruit and eggs. One overly exuberant reveller sent a hot ember caroming off His Majesty's cranium, toasting to a turn portions of the royal skull and face and leaving several unsightly scars. Displaying the sort of ingenuity worthy of a fun-loving king, Francis grew a beard to hide the disfigurement, and his loyal subjects soon followed suit. Not to be outdone by a mere Frenchman, Henry VIII promptly sprouted his famous furry frame, and the fashion was firmly entrenched on both sides of the Channel. Small wonder that monarchism is on the wane: life at the palace simply is not what it used to be.

Religious Beards

The church, which throughout history has always regarded most things with greater sobriety than has the Crown, was no less serious about beards.

Scripture specifically prohibits shaving: "They shall not make baldness upon their head, neither shall they shave off the corner of their beard, nor make any cuttings in their flesh" (Leviticus 21:5). Inasmuch as the reference is specifically to shaving, many Orthodox Jews use chemical depilatories or electric razors, which do not "make any cuttings in their flesh." The beard is nevertheless still a symbol of patriarchy, scholarliness, and veneration. II Samuel 10:4 and Isaiah 7:20, 50:6 relate that "any mutilation

41

or insult to the beard was considered a mortal disgrace" (*Universal Jewish Encyclopedia*, Vol. II; New York, 1948), an attitude which continued in effect for some time. The soon-to-be King John, visiting Ireland in 1185, "gave deadly offence" to the Irish chieftains by pulling their beards.

Hebraic reverence for the beard persists in other religions. Muslims continue to swear by the beard of the Prophet. Mohammed ordered his disciples to grow beards so that they might be distinguished from Christians, but to trim them so as to avoid being mistaken for Jews.

Shaving and beard-trimming are considered signs of vanity in the Eastern Orthodox

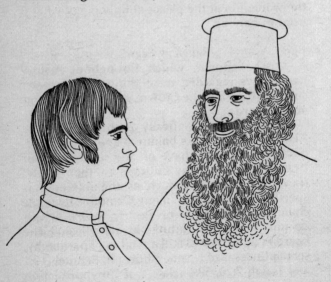

churches ("An Oral Dissertation on the Customs of Eastern Orthodoxy" by G. Touloumes; 1971, New York: Jarrow Press, Inc.). Beards were in fact one of the issues in the Great Schism (1378-1417), resulting in the general beardlessness of the Roman clergy and the full, glorious beards of the Eastern clergy.

Publius Lentulus, who preceded Herod as proconsul of Judea, sent the following description as part of a report to the Roman Senate:

> ". . . At this time appeared a man who is still living and endowed with mighty power; his name is Jesus Christ . . . the hair of his head is the colour of wine. . . . His beard is abundant, the same colour as the hair, and forked . . ." (A. N. Didron, *Christian Iconography*, 1886; republished 1965 by Frederick Ungar Publishing Co., New York).

A now-obscure but once-important group of 19th century Roman artists who called themselves the Nazarenes were the first to depict Jesus with the long wavy hair and rather thin beard with which we are so familiar today. It is "a curiously sentimental interpretation," declares art commentator Russell Lynes, "of a very decidedly tough-minded philosopher."

A *Byzantine Guide to Painting* (Didron, *op. cit.*), which first appeared sometime in the 15th or 16th century, was very specific about the depiction of Biblical figures. Adam, Cain, and Abel are described as beardless. (A Romanesque column in Spain shows Adam as smooth-chinned before The Fall and bearded afterward.) But beardlessness in the *Guide* is synonymous with youth; later on, the Holy Patriarchs are

43

all bewhiskered: "Adam: an old man, long hair, white beard. . . . Noah: an old man, beard pointed. . . . Shem, son of Noah: . . . beard bifurcated [forked]. . . . Abraham: . . . long hair, beard descending to his waist. . . . The righteous Simeon, who received the Lord in his arms: an old man, great beard." The *Guide* contains many lines on the painting of the Trinity, with meticulous and lengthy instructions for representing God the Father, God the Son (both bearded, of course), and the Holy Spirit.

Artistic Beards

Even during those periods when beards were out of fashion, it was not unusual for men in the arts to wear them. Sprouting chins were —and, in some quarters, still are—regarded as emblematic of *la vie bohème*. Shakespeare, Dostoevski, Tolstoi, Walt Whitman, Robert Browning, Hemingway, Longfellow, D. H. Lawrence, Johannes Brahms, Sir Adrian Boult, Ernest Ansermet, Sir Thomas Beecham, Mitch Miller, Burl Ives, Skitch Henderson, Van Gogh, Monet, Manet, Degas, Renoir, Monty Woolley, Peter Ustinov, Sebastian Cabot, Vincent Price, Orson Welles, are but a handful of artists with concealed chins. But perhaps the most famous literary beard of our century was the formidable one worn by George Bernard Shaw.

Some Other Famous Beards

Beards have been perpetuated in glory and in infamy. Frederick I, King of Prussia (1152), was known as Frederick Barbarossa, or "Redbeard," while the Chevalier Raoul lives forever in the folklore of crime as "Bluebeard," whose seventh wife happened upon the remains of her six less fortunate predecessors.

Any list of famous beards must include those of William ("Trade") and Andrew ("Mark") Smith, the brothers who built a commercial colossus on the foundations of their father's cough

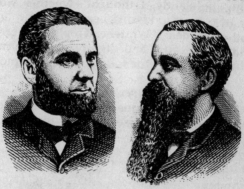

drop business which they inherited in 1872. The brothers were of stern Scottish stock; and "Trade," by far the more domineering of the pair, was a strict prohibitionist as well as an openhanded philanthropist. He demonstrates both virtues by donating a park in Poughkeepsie, N.Y. (the firm's home since its founding), with the proviso that if liquor were ever sold on the property, the land would revert to the family. As though standing guard to insure that his edict is obeyed, "Trade" Smith's somber bearded countenance gazes down from a monument high on a hill in the park.

The most easily recognized beard in America today belongs, paradoxically, to an

Englishman: Commander Edward Whitehead, C.B.E., chairman of the board of Schweppes USA Ltd. Some years ago, when Jack Paar was still host of the *Tonight Show* television program, the Commander appeared as a guest. A young starlet, whose name has mercifully slipped from memory, asked the Commander—rather petulantly, I thought—whether women did not object to kissing bearded men.

"My dear," Whitehead replied, a veritable pillar of elegance and dignity, "no one minds going through a little foliage to get to a picnic."

The Superlative Beard
If a youth begins shaving at the age of 15, he is likely to dispose of some nine yards of

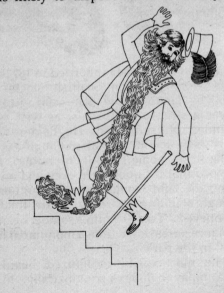

whiskers in his lifetime and expend about 3,350 hours — the equivalent of approximately 139 days — at the task.

Among those who considered such labors as wasteful was Hans Steininger, distinguished burgomaster of Braunau, Austria, whose beard was over eight feet long. In 1567, Herr Steininger, doubtlessly preoccupied with the cares of office, tripped over his beard, plummetted down a flight of stairs, and met his untimely end.

The *Guinness Book of World Records* (New York: 1971 [Revised Edition]: Sterling Publishing Co., Inc.) informs that the longest beard ever recorded belonged to Hans Langreth. Born in Norway in 1846, Langreth emigrated to the United States where he died in 1927, leaving behind a beard measuring $17\frac{1}{2}$ feet. In 1967, the beard was presented to the Smithsonian Institution in Washington. I have no idea where, how, or by whom it was cared for in the intervening years.

Despite the vagaries of custom and the vicissitudes of history, one fact stands out with diamondlike clarity: the beard has always been a symbol of manhood and virility. The artist, the poet, the sculptor — and woman — have all paid tribute to beards through the ages; and though transient, fickle fashion may dictate the temporary discontinuance of facial growth, beards always return, for it is only natural that they should do so.

If God had wanted you to have a hairless chin, He would have given you one.

3. A GLOSSARY OF THE BEARD

Beards come in as many styles and variations as there are faces on which to grow them. No beard looks exactly the same on two different people, which is as it should be; the beard is a distinguishing mark of a man and deserves the distinction of individuality.

In Chapter 5 we shall discuss the selection of a beard best suited to you; but before doing so, it is necessary that you become acquainted, in a general way, with some of the more common varieties of beards. Bear in mind that, despite the generalities, your beard will be distinctly and individually yours.

This listing is not alphabetical because many of the designations are arbitrary, and therefore an alphabetical list would serve no purpose. Some of the designations, in fact, were created specifically for this book. In any case, this glossary is intended for use not as a dictionary but as a guide to various types of beards, generally beginning with the fullest, and progressing—or regressing, depending on one's viewpoint—to the meagerest, pausing along the way for variations in style.

HIPPIE-FREAKIE

This is literally a case of "letting it all hang out." The beard is allowed to grow, willy-nilly, without guidance, cultivation, or topiary of any kind. It may grow in a variety of directions, covering all points of the compass. De-

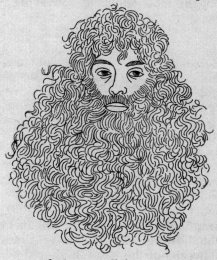

pending on their overall hirsute propensities, Hippie-Freakie beard wearers may find hair growing from directly beneath the eyes, *i.e.*, high up on the cheekbones. The Hippie-Freakie suggests a certain looseness of life style and is not recommended for persons engaged in somewhat restrictive pursuits, such as banking or marriage counseling.

RABBINICAL/EASTERN ORTHODOX

The primary difference between this somewhat ecclesiastical style and the Hippie-Freakie is that the Rabbinical/Eastern Orthodox (R/EO) is meticulously washed and carefully combed. Where the Hippie-Freakie tends to become even more entangled in a high wind, the R/EO floats, gossamerlike, on the breeze.

Of all the various types of beards, the R/EO is the most strokable, conveying a truly

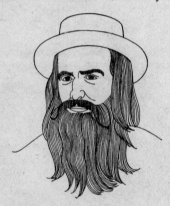

imposing image of sagacity as its wearer thoughtfully caresses it with long, almost sensuous sweeps of the hand. It should be noted that the R/EO is hardly ever trimmed or cut. It is, however, constantly combed and brushed, if not with actual barbering tools, then with the palm and fingers.

The R/EO is one of the most beautiful specimens in all of beard-dom. It should be reserved for clergymen, dedicated scholars, and ascetics.

FULL BEARD

Here, too, the beard is allowed to grow at will, sprouting from any point on the face where it happens to flourish. The primary difference is that the Full Beard is cut. While the two previously described beards are allowed to grow and grow, the Full Beard is trimmed and clipped, usually rather close to the face. It is a style well suited to those who wish to appear professorial, medical, or scientific. Louis Pasteur and Sigmund Freud both wore beards of this type.

PARTIAL-FULL BEARD

This seeming contradiction in terms is actually something of a small deception. On some men, a full beard constitutes a rather heavy growth, covering a large area. Sometimes, for purely cosmetic purposes, it is desirable to shave a bit under the eyes and high up on the cheeks, directly below the lower lip, or on either side of the little tuft of hair which grows just under the lower lip. The overall effect is that of the Full Beard. Actually, however, there has been some trimming. The author wears a Partial-Full Beard.

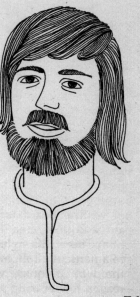

PENNSYLVANIA DUTCH

More properly, this style should be attributed to the Amish sect which, while proliferating in Pennsylvania, can be found in great numbers in other parts of the United States, notably Ohio. Amishmen adhere to the Biblical injunction against shaving, and a man is expected to let his beard grow when he marries.

The Amish are pacifists and refuse to associate themselves with anything which even remotely smacks of the military. As a result they do not wear buttons on their clothes, nor do they wear mustaches, which at one time were the trademark of the European soldier.

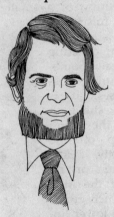

The beard is usually cut straight across at the bottom, creating a somewhat stolid effect. I have seen this style on men who do not belong to a particular religious sect but who merely like the way it looks, which is perhaps the best reason for wearing any kind of beard.

LINCOLNESQUE

This is something of a combination between the Full and the Pennsylvania Dutch, in that it requires shaving the upper lip. Men who choose to wear a Lincolnesque would do well to remember the stature—historical as well as physical—of the man with whom it is most closely associated.

It is yet another commentary on the infinite wisdom of the feminine mind that President Lincoln's beard was inspired by a female. Shortly after the election of 1860, Grace Bedell, age 11, wrote to Lincoln suggesting he grow a beard. The president-elect replied: "As to the

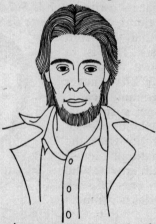

whiskers, having never worn any, do you not think people would call it a piece of silly affection [sic] if I were to begin it now?" Nevertheless, a photograph taken about a month prior to the inauguration shows Mr. Lincoln with the now-famous whiskers.

RING-FRAME

This style can perhaps best be described as a close-cropped Lincolnesque. It consists of a ring of short hair, issuing from the sideburns in a continuous line around the face. It is cut perfectly evenly on all sides and forms a circular frame; hence its name.

For reasons I am unable to explain, I have always associated the Ring-Frame with sternness and austerity, two qualities which tend to put me off. I have no doubt that some very amiable, openhanded people, perhaps even a hedonist here and there, wear the Ring-Frame. Nevertheless, whenever I see one, I instantly assume that its owner spends Sundays reading the Bible aloud, disapproves of dancing, and is unaware that the word "sex" exists. This is, of course, pure conjecture on my part. I have never met a Ring-Frame wearer, which is not surprising. Having the kinds of associations I do with the style, I naturally avoid contact with anyone who has grown one. Of such vicious cycles is paranoia born.

It is, therefore, with complete subjectivity that I suggest that the Ring-Frame be worn by dedicated missionaries, farmers in very cold climates, prohibitionists, and celibates who have dedicated their lives to the dubious and doomed cause of universal virginity.

54

VANDYKE

Properly, this should be spelled Van Dyck, after the Flemish painter; but purists who insist on the Dutch spelling will also have to demand the retention of the original style to which the Old Master gave his name, and therein lies trouble. Perhaps no other type of beard has so many variations.

Basically, the Vandyke is a chin beard. Its sides tend to be parallel with the corners of the mouth and the beard itself is relatively short. (A long Vandyke is more accurately called a Goatee, *q.v.*) But any attempt to describe accurately what are today called Vandykes must end there. Some have rounded or ovate bottoms; others are cut square across; still others terminate in dirklike points. The top of the beard, i.e., that portion which is directly beneath the lower lip, is subject to as many variations as the bottom. Some are allowed to grow naturally; others are scooped out, creating the impression of a cup made of hair; still others are shaped and carved with topiary craftsmanship. Thus it may be safely assumed that any short beard which covers most of the chin can be termed a Vandyke or a variation thereof.

Vandykes are in evidence everywhere, for they cover a multitude of needs and circumstances. It is, for example, an enormous advantage to a psychiatrist, enabling him to raise his fees by some 20%. If, in addition, he can produce a Viennese accent, the sky is the limit. However, while the beard with the accent is a winning combination, the beard *without* the accent will also serve well, whereas the accent

55

without the beard may very well label even the most competent of practitioners as nothing more than an opportunistic, upstart foreigner.

Physicians, chiropodists, chiropractors, osteopaths, pharmacists, barbers, hairdressers, busboys—in short, anyone whose profession entitles him to wear a white coat—would do well to consider growing a Vandyke; thanks to television commercials and magazine advertisements, the combined effect of the white coat and the beard lends an aura of professionalism unmatched by any other appurtenance, except possibly a stethoscope casually protruding from one's pocket. (This device, however, could be regarded as something of an affectation at, say, the opera or a cocktail party, while the beard, permanently attached and always in evidence, is quite acceptable.)

Even a dentist can wear a Vandyke. In fact, this is probably the only kind of beard a dentist should consider at all, as many patients seem somewhat querulous about having a large quantity of someone else's hair so close to their open mouths.

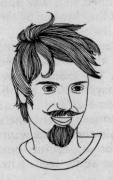

If I had to nominate a universal beard, it would be the Vandyke. It greatly enhances the physiognomies of men in prestigious positions, while at the same time elevating the personal status of those in somewhat lowlier occupations. The Vandyke serves the additional purpose of affording the would-be pogonotropher the opportunity of beginning with a small but nonetheless presentable beard from which he may ultimately expand into wider pastures . . . in a manner of speaking.

GOATEE

This is an unfortunate designation for a not-unattractive beard. Goatees closely resemble the beards worn by goats; hence the name. For an excellent example of what a proper goatee should look like, the reader is advised to inspect

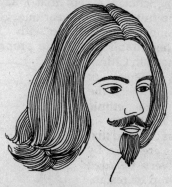

a goat. A billy goat, of course. Caution should be observed, however, as those who have inspected billy goats too closely have often reported discomfiting consequences.

Goatees are especially handsome when they are white and accompanied by flowing white hair. Other useful accessories for setting off a Goatee to best advantage are: a string tie, a mint julep, and a pillared mansion in a state of decrepitude.

ORIENTAL SCHOLAR

Orientals generally have rather sparse facial hair. Most oriental beards, therefore, are thin and wispy. But what they lack in body is compensated for in length. The result is a longish beard, somewhat resembling a Goatee, but considerably thinner. The Oriental Scholar beard is always accompanied by a long, drooping mustache.

There is no reason, I suppose, why this type of beard cannot be called simply Oriental, without the Scholar, except that I have never seen anyone but a scholar wear one. Given my somewhat meager intercourse with Orientals, confined — regrettably — largely to proprietors of souvenir shops in China- town and owners of restaurants in which the most exquisite ethnic cuisine flourishes, I nevertheless contend that such beards are worn by scholars. Every bearded souvenir shop or restau- rant owner I have ever seen was always im- mersed in a book, and it was clear from the ex-

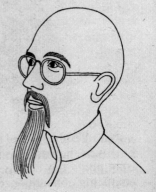

pressions on their faces that they were not reading anything frivolous.

An interesting sidelight is that Occidentals who wear Oriental Scholar beards soon become Orientalized (not to be confused with *oriented* which is a business and military expression, or *orientated*, which is a linguistic abomination). An acquaintance of mine, a computer programmer, is a middle-aged gentleman of Eastern European ancestry. He grew an Oriental Scholar beard and has since learned to speak Chinese. He is at times mistaken for a Jewish mandarin.

UNDERLIP

Almost all men with any quantity of facial hair will find, if they refrain from shaving for a few days, that a small tuft of hair will appear directly beneath the center of the lower lip. If this is left to flourish while the rest of the face is shaved, the result will be the Underlip, known in bygone days as the *mouche*, a style very popular among the French and Dutch cavaliers who peer out from ancestral portraits and from cigar boxes. In recent years, it has become known as the "bop beard," popularized by jazz musician Dizzy Gillespie. The Underlip has proliferated in the black community, possibly as a tribute to that most talented and accomplished soul brother.

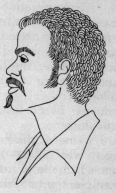

There is a certain restrained raffishness associated with the Underlip, a man-of-the-worldish, screw-you-I'm-all-right-Jack attitude. They are, in the current vernacular, very cool. I always believe that Underlip wearers engage only in activities at which they excel and that such activities are always enviable. If you have business with old ladies, I would advise you to avoid the Underlip. If, on the other hand, you have business with *young* ladies, I am convinced that the Underlip can be instrumental in helping you to progress to social intercourse—at least.

There is one small group of Underlip wearers which constitutes an exception to the above generalization. Certain nervous types grow Underlips in order to have something convenient to chew on. While this is healthier than chain-smoking and less puerile than nail-biting, it is nevertheless a disgusting habit.

MEPHISTOPHELIAN

The operative word here is: Points. The beard itself ends in a sharp point; its sides, usually unconnected, are trimmed so that very sharp angles are displayed, and the portion directly under the lip is cut to resemble three pikes, separated by perfectly symmetrical valleys.

A blond or gray Mephistophelian is ridiculous.

The Mephistophelian should be worn by a man with at least one or two Satanic propensities which he is interested in advertising. For example, the two Mephistophelians with which

I have had contact belong to men of completely divergent personalities; yet the style suits them both perfectly. One, an author, instantly creates an impression of inherent nastiness. One expects him to be hostile, vitriolic, demanding, and unreasonable, and one is therefore not surprised when he proves to be all of these things.

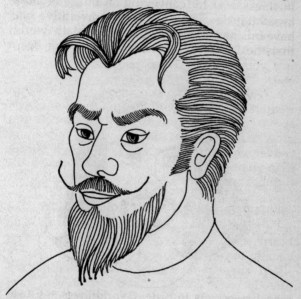

The other is a gentleman of almost unctuous charm who oozes lechery. Not surprisingly, he is a senior editor for a publisher of pornography.

If you wear a Mephistophelian beard, people—especially women—will be distrustful of you. Depending on your goals, this is not necessarily a disadvantage.

RING BEARD

The beard (kept very short) and the mustache form an almost perfect circle around the lips, framing the mouth.

This style is recommended for men who believe they have particularly attractive mouths and wish to emphasize them. The Ring Beard is also useful for conveying an image of close-mouthedness. The effect is a provocative one: a beard, any beard, suggests a certain worldliness; it follows, therefore, that a Ring Beard

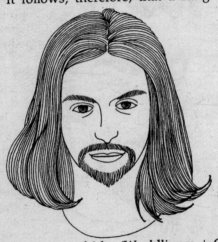

man has secrets to hide. (Worldliness + Close-mouthedness = Secrets.) Attempts to pry those secrets loose can result in some fascinating social activity.

A word of caution: cigar smokers should avoid this style. The combination of the phallic-looking cigar and the Ring Beard results in a picture which can only be described as obscene.

MISCELLANEOUS TOPIARY

Were you to peruse a standard barbering text (which task I have already performed for you), you would find such beard names as Anchor, French Fork, Tailored Fork, Old Dutch, Flat Bottom, Long Vandyke with Exposed Chin, etc. While such terms may serve some purpose for the professional, they only tend to confuse the amateur pogonotropher.

Topiary is defined in *Webster's Seventh New Collegiate Dictionary* as ". . . the practice or art of training, cutting, and trimming trees or shrubs into odd or ornamental shapes. . . ." Any pogonophile knows that the practice is by no means confined to the shrubbery in the garden.

As a generally conservative man who appreciates tradition, I tend to avoid fancy, overly ornate or patently outlandish hirsute topiary. At the same time, I respect every man's right to free himself of inhibition as long as he is aware of the possible consequences and is prepared to meet them. If you feel comfortable with a chin which looks as though someone had pasted a miniature hairy anchor to it, who am I to gainsay your right to grow such a beard? After all, it is your face. Do with it what you will.

4. HAIRY ANCILLARIES

Careful attention must be paid by the would-be pogonotropher to mustache and sideburns. He must first consider whether he wishes to cultivate them, and second, if so, he must decide what kind he will grow. Proper matching is as important to one's face as it is to one's wardrobe. A full, flowing, luxuriant beard accompanied by a mere snippet of a brush beneath the nose is about as appropriate as a cutaway coat, striped trousers, and tennis shoes.

There is no precise, prescribed combination of mustaches, sideburns, and beards. While certain combinations, as just mentioned, are completely ridiculous, there is nevertheless considerable leeway, and serious thought must be given to the shape of the face, the height and weight of the wearer, the image one wishes to convey, the growth pattern of facial hair, etc. Bear in mind, too, that the more skin is covered by hair, the less shaving one must endure— surely an advantage not to be lightly passed over. (See *Making the Connection*, below.)

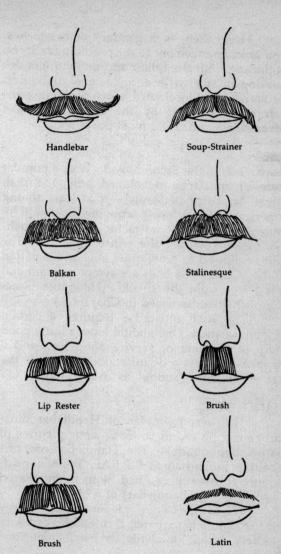

Handlebar

Soup-Strainer

Balkan

Stalinesque

Lip Rester

Brush

Brush

Latin

Here, then, is a glossary of mustaches, similar in arrangement to the preceding chapter; beginning with the fullest and more or less decreasing in size, with an occasional digression for variations. Once more, much of the nomenclature is invented by the author, but will nevertheless suffice for most purposes.

RAF

During the Second World War, a popular style of mustache developed among British Royal Air Force personnel—or at least among American film actors portraying British RAF personnel. The RAF mustache is a large, brush-like affair, covering the entire upper lip. The hair is allowed to grow quite long and is parted in the middle. The ends are swept outward and stand free from the cheeks. (How this is accomplished is discussed in Chapter 8.)

The RAF mustache requires a certain amount of dash. One should have a fairly good store of wartime or service anecdotes, and a clipped accent is a definite asset. Cultivate the use of the word "ruddy" as an adjective.

HANDLEBAR

The best examples of Handlebar mustaches can be found in *fin-de-siècle* pictures of barbershop quartets. The Handlebar contains about as much hair as the RAF. The major difference is that it is combed, shaped, and waxed to resemble the handlebars of a bicycle.

The mustache cup was invented primarily for the Handlebar wearer. It resembles ordinary crockery, except for a wide, flat barrier along one side of the top. The barrier lifts the mustache up and away from the liquid, which pours through an opening at the lower part of the barrier. It is obvious that unless one exercises extreme care, Handlebar mustaches can be a mess, only a shade less sloppy than the Soup-Strainer (*q.v.*).

The Handlebar is admittedly an old-fashioned style, which seems to go with straw boaters, hair parted in the middle, and striped bathing costumes. Nevertheless, it can be carried off with considerable aplomb by certain men, especially when accompanied by a Full or Partial-Full beard. The most important factor is attitude. The Handlebar must be worn with complete confidence and with a display of gentlemanly but unmistakable disdain for those who would snicker. If you find yourself apologizing for a Handlebar, it is the wrong style for you.

SOUP-STRAINER

The Soup-Strainer is essentially a Handlebar which droops. It is suitable only for supremely fastidious eaters or those who are customarily fed intravenously.

The Soup-Strainer is highly recommended for men who wish to remain celibate but are reluctant to advertise such preference, since it greatly inhibits and discourages kissing. It is likely to deposit a quantity of hair into the mouth of the kissee and often gives off an effluvium reminiscent of the kisser's last two or three meals. It may even retain a morsel or two of food. Such conditions have been known to curtail sexual activities.

BALKAN

Now we come to the first of the cropped mustaches. The Balkan is a wide band of hair completely covering the upper lip and extending somewhat beyond the corners of the mouth. Cropped fairly close to the skin, this style is favored by Greeks, Turks, an occasional Bulgarian, and others around whom an aura of international intrigue and dark mystery prevails.

The Balkan is an excellent style of mustache for men with long, sharp features and/or small mouths. If not exaggerated, the Balkan will work wonders at bringing the face into better symmetry and balance. I wore one for years before growing my beard.

STALINESQUE

The Stalinesque is a variation of the Balkan, distinguished by little points at the bottoms of the outer edges. It is a good design for men with somewhat round, soft-featured faces, as it provides some additional angularity. Stalinesque wearers should avoid the company of virulent patriots with good memories.

BRUSH

This single term covers a wide variety of mustache types, all of which have two features in common: (1) They cover the entire width of the upper lip, from just under the nose to where the lip itself begins. (2) They never extend beyond the corners of the mouth.

For some men, there is little difference between the Brush and the Balkan. For others, the Brush can be just a smidgen of hair under the nose. Brushes are much favored by accountants, civil servants, older male librarians, and male nurses—in short, by men who feel the need to assert either their maleness or their maturity (sometimes, alas, both) but who are conservative by nature. Yes, the Brush is almost always worn by conservative men.

There are, of course, exceptions. There is one style of Brush which is about an inch-and-a-half wide. If you elect to wear this type, never let your hair fall over your right forehead. Avoid Jewish neighborhoods.

LIP RESTER

Any mustache which uses the upper lip as its base and which does not extend beyond the outer edges of the lip qualifies as a Lip Rester, whether it be thick or thin, narrow or wide. But note: if it reaches the nose, it becomes a Brush.

The Lip Rester is highly recommended for men with thick lips.

LATIN

With great care and patience, and a steady hand, it is possible to shape a mustache *in the middle* of the area between the nose and the lip. Experts have managed to create such mustaches which look as though they were drawn with a pencil. For some reason, probably connected with the terrible films with which I wasted my mind in the 30's and 40's, I always associate such mustaches with so-called Latin types; hence the name. In later years, I came to relate the style to disreputable used car salesmen, white slavers, professional gamblers, and men who sell protection. This is, of course, utter nonsense.

Men who grow Latin mustaches should learn to tango.

MISCELLANEOUS

As with beards, the shape and style of the mustache depends greatly on the individual wearer. Combinations and variations of styles are always in evidence. Ben Turpin, the great silent film comedian, displayed the most magnificent example of Brush-Soup-Strainer combination ever seen in public. Avoid stereotypes and rigid definitions. Experiment; find the style which suits you best.

Some Notes about Sideburns

Not too long ago, it was a simple matter to define sideburns: the hair which grows along the side of the face, in front of the ears. Now, however, with longer sideburns in fashion, the definition becomes less clear. If you were to draw an imaginary line from the bottom of your ear lobe, extending under and parallel with your eye, you would most likely mark off the approximate line at which your beard begins growing. Technically, then, *anything which grows below that line is a beard.* If it is strictly a vertical extension of your natural sideburns, then it probably qualifies as a sideburn. If, however, it extends into the area of the cheek, is it or is it not a sideburn? That could depend on how wide the strip of hair or how narrow the cheek; whether the sideburn is attached to a

70

mustache or a beard; whether it extends clear down to the jaw line, etc., etc. As you can see, the whole question of defining sideburns bids fair to become extremely complex.

Therefore, my advice to you is: forget it. What is of primary concern is how you look and feel. As a pogonotropher, you require a certain amount of free spirit. Do not allow yourself to become bogged down by nomenclature and precise specification, which in any case will rapidly deteriorate into virtually unintelligible jargon (*vide* any standard text on sociology or education).

Making the Connection

Whether sideburns, mustache, and beard should be connected depends on individual taste and appearance. It might be wise, however, to keep in mind that when any segments of the total beard are unconnected, there is exposed skin which must be shaved at more or less regular intervals. You will be pleased to learn that even if this is the case, it may not be necessary to shave as often as you did when you were beardless. In my own case, I have been able to progress from shaving daily—sometimes, under special circumstances, *twice* daily—to shaving every other day. Even then, it takes me half the time it used to take. The reason is obvious: when whiskers begin to sprout on an unbearded face, they are very much in evidence. A beard, however, is sufficiently dark to provide the necessary contrast between the bearded and unbearded areas to mitigate the slight shadow on the exposed skin.

An important factor to consider is your condition when shaving. If you are, perforce, a morning shaver and if, like me, you are groggy, grouchy, and usually late, it is best not to have to contend with too many borderlines and boundaries. A clean-shaven man need only rake his face with the blade, pray that he will not perish from exsanguination, and make his way to his morning transfusion of caffeine. A bearded man with unconnected mustache and/or sideburns, however, must exercise great care. He must be alert and meticulous. Few things look more pathetic than a lopsided, uneven beard or mustache. Any attempt to even out the edges in the morning usually ends in disaster. Many is the Balkan that has been reduced to a Brush; many is the Vandyke that has been frantically trimmed to an Underlip. I speak from painful personal experience. This is, in fact, the major contributing factor in my graduating from a Vandyke to a Partial-Full.

Now that you know the history of beards and have a store of other fascinating facts, now that you have become acquainted with some of the more typical styles, the time has come at last: you are ready to choose a beard of your very own.

5. SELECTING A BEARD

I began shaving at the age of 14. During the ensuing 10 years, I made several abortive attempts to grow a mustache, but whenever I tried, I ended up looking like the kind of fellow who used to carry a black suitcase and sidle up to you on the sidewalk with an offer to sell you rubber goods and illicit comic books. Some of my more outspoken friends claimed that I resembled a Spanish pimp (which, secretly, I took as a compliment; the sobriquet, however, played havoc with my social standing). Quite by accident, I eventually discovered why I was having trouble growing a presentable mustache, and in the process happened upon a technique for beard selection which is virtually foolproof. (It is fitting that this happy event occurred while I was in college, a place which nowadays seems less and less suited for learning much of anything, either by accident or design.)

I was loitering in the office of the college newspaper, leafing through a copy of the latest edition, which bore a small portrait of me at the top of a column which I wrote. Idly I began to doodle, and drew a mustache on my upper lip. It turned out to be a Balkan and I saw, with the clarity of one who attains *satori*, that this was the mustache for me. It took approximately two-and-a-half weeks to grow one and I have had it ever since, modifying it slightly to accommodate my beard, which was added later. At the same time, I devised a means of beard selection which I now pass on to you. Pay close attention; this may well be the most important part of this book.

Beard selection should not be a hit-and-miss proposition. To experiment on your face is time-consuming and, unless you have the great good fortune to hit upon the right style the first time, the results can be anything from frustrating to ludicrous. (Note: there is nothing wrong with experimenting *after* you have developed your basic beard. See Chapter 10.) Of course, you could acquire a quantity of false beards and then attempt to duplicate the one you like best; but this might prove not only expensive, but well-nigh impossible in many communities without expending considerable time and effort. Take heart — there is a way.

No matter where you live, there is, somewhere nearby, a vending machine which takes pictures. You know the kind I mean. You sit inside a little booth, draw the curtain for privacy, insert a coin, watch for the flashing light, and *voilà!* In minutes, your impressive countenance is disgorged, in quadruplicate, from a chute. You can find these booths at amusement parks, railway and bus terminals, airports, or at your local five-and-ten. Seek out such a booth and have your picture taken, making sure that you wind up with the following poses: full face serious, full face smiling, left profile, and right profile.

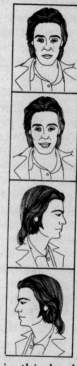

Your next stop is an art supply dealer or a good stationery store. Purchase a large sheet of clear acetate and a black or brown china marker, which is a crayonlike pencil expressly designed to write on hard, glossy surfaces (such as china). It is sometimes called a grease pencil. Buy only black or brown, regardless of the color of your beard. Red or yellow china markers bear no resemblance to actual hair color. If you live in an area racked by runaway inflation, you will have spent as much as three dollars and are now fully prepared to engage in beard selection.

Study the illustrations in this book and select the beard types which appeal to you most. Also study live beards, those belonging to people you know or see on television, as well as beards in magazines and newspapers, etc. Now, lay the acetate sheet over your pictures and, with the china marker, *draw the beard and mustache you like best*. Be sure to draw it over all four pictures. If you make a mistake, simply rub off the china marker with ordinary facial tissue and start again.

After you have drawn a beard to your satisfaction, lift the acetate sheet—carefully, to avoid smudging your artwork—and place it down again, with an unmarked area over the pictures, and start all over, this time with a different style. Repeat the process as often as you like, until you have drawn all the styles you think are worthy of your consideration.

This is the time to give free rein to your imagination. Try all the beard/mustache/sideburns combinations which come to mind and which you feel will look attractive. Even try a few which you think are silly, or ill-suited; you may well be surprised at the results. A stroke of the marker connects sideburns to mustache; a swipe of the facial tissue disconnects them again. Sweep the ends of the mustache up, turn them down, stick them straight out. Give yourself an Underlip, a bifurcated Vandyke, a Mutton Chop, a Ring-Frame. Keep switching from one set of drawings to another, "trying on" each one to see which looks best.

(If you have the time and inclination for frivolity, take out the family album and, using the acetate sheet, bestow an assortment of whiskers on your relatives and friends. Mothers-in-law in particular seem to take on a different aspect when secretly bearded and are frequently much easier to cope with afterward. It would be imprudent, however, to let the dear lady know about the liberties you have taken with her face. As a matter of fact, you may run the risk of discovering a deficiency in your wife's sense of humor at this point. In any event, do not allow this admittedly puerile exercise to deter you from your original purpose.)

In Chapter 7 we shall examine at length how to deal with the obstacles to pogonotrophy which will be thrust in your path by various people. However, it is not premature at this juncture to discuss what may prove to be your most formidable opposition: The Woman in Your Life. For simplicity's sake, we shall assume that she is your wife, with the understanding that she could as easily be your mother, daughter, secretary, fiancée, paramour, or landlady. Only one of these stands out above the others—unless you are indeed a man among men or a congenital liar—and therefore only that one needs to be won over to pogonotrophy. Otherwise, she will either deter you or make your life miserable.

Invite your wife to join you in the Acetate-over-the-Picture Beard Selection Technique. If she is committed to the idea of your wearing a beard she will prove quite useful, exercising the cold objectivity of which women are capable when it comes to passing judgment on men. If, on the other hand, she is firmly set against the whole proposition, appeal to her sense of fair play by asking that she at least look at the pictures. You will find that she is soon participating, making suggestions and recommendations, and, finally, saying something like: "Well, I think *that* one looks best." *Hooked!* She has unwittingly committed herself by participating and by expressing her preference. Chapter 7 will help you proceed from there, but for really difficult cases, ask your local librarian to recommend a good text on salesmanship.

When selecting a beard, keep in mind all that has been discussed in previous chapters. Remember that a number of elements enter into your choice:

The size of the face: A small face will disappear under a mass of hair. You will find it difficult to win the respect of your family, friends, and colleagues if all they see is a mat with nothing but a nose sticking out of it, except for an occasional hole which appears to ingest food and drink or to make conversation. Similarly, a small beard on a large face will look as though you had missed a spot while shaving. Prudence, Brother, prudence. To exaggerate is to invite ridicule.

The shape of the face: A beard can work miracles in correcting facial flaws or in en-

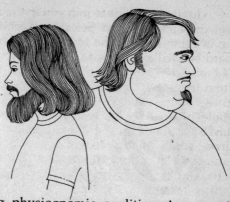

hancing physiognomic qualities. A man with a weak, receding chin can strengthen his features by growing a beard, just as a face with a strong, well-defined jawline can be enhanced by a beard which accentuates that quality. It is essential that you select the type of beard which complements your features. For example, *a sharply pointed beard* improves a somewhat round face, creating the impression of elongation. It should never be worn on an angular, thin, or long face. *A rounded beard* softens angularity, shortens a longish chin, but exaggerates a round or fleshy face. *A squarish beard* will relieve the lines of a triangular face. *A wide beard* will help round out an oval face. *A narrow beard* will help elongate a round face, provided the beard is not too narrow.

Social and professional considerations also enter into beard selection. Despite my frequent declarations that pogonotrophy is synonymous with individuality, there are limits, and it is wise to stay within the guidelines estab-

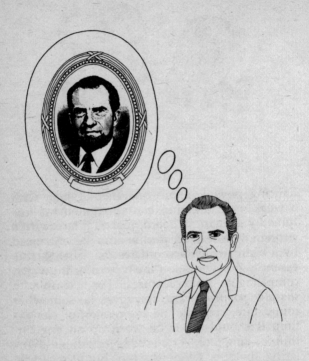

lished by your job or profession and by the social milieu in which you prefer to circulate. There is a vast difference between being individualistic and making a spectacle of yourself.

When you have at last decided on the beard you want, draw the style directly on to the pictures. You are now ready to begin cultivating your very own beard on your very own face.

Grow forth.

6. PLOTTING THE BEARD

The prime requisite for plotting a beard is hair. It will therefore be necessary for you to allow your beard to grow a little. I recommend that you skip at least three regular shaves before beginning. Some men may be obliged to skip as many as four or five shaves, depending upon the thickness and color of growth. Please note that I have said *shaves*, and not days. In other words, if you normally shave every day, you can begin shaping your beard on the fourth day, but if you shave only twice a week, you will have some difficulty unless you wait until well into the second week of nonshaving.

Be prepared to defend yourself. People's attitudes toward bristly chins range from slight revulsion to smart-alecky wisecracking and you will encounter them all. How to handle yourself in various situations which arise at this time will be discussed in the next chapter, but one cannot prepare too early to stand up for one's rights.

You will require the following implements:

An eyebrow pencil the approximate color
of your beard.

A sharp razor.

A good mirror which you can get quite
close to. A magnifying mirror is ideal.

Hot, almost scalding, water.

A clear eye.

A steady hand.

THE EYEBROW PENCIL

You will need an eyebrow pencil to outline the contours of your beard and, for a short
time, to fill in uneven spots. Ask your wife or
girlfriend to lend you one. If she claims that she
has none to spare, she is lying. There is not a
woman alive in the United States who uses cosmetics who does not have an excess of them.

If you are unable to appropriate one, buy
one at the drug or department store. You should
be able to get one for about 50 cents. Do not
allow the clerk to con you into the more expensive varieties, which are designed to convince
women that ostentatious packaging and su-
perfluous mechanics are worth paying for.

Some men are embarrassed at the pros-
pect of buying an eyebrow pencil for themselves. This is foolish. If you are married and
have suffered through the ordeal of picking up
tampons or sanitary napkins for your wife, there
is nothing in the druggist's stock which ought
to faze you. Remember that the salesperson's
sole purpose in life is to provide you with merchandise in exchange for money — *your* money.
There is no reason why this stranger, whom
you will probably never see again, should in-

timidate you. If you must, you can always mumble something about a part in the church play. You will not be believed, but it may make you feel better.

THE RAZOR

If you use a safety razor, insert a new blade before you begin beard-shaping. You will be pleasantly surprised to learn that your longer facial hairs are much easier to shave because (a) they are softer and (b) it is easier for the blade to get a good purchase on them. Nevertheless, there may be an occasional snag which can prove slightly painful and can, therefore, throw you off. A new blade should prevent such an occurrence.

I do not recommend the use of an electric shaver for beard-shaping because I find it difficult to do fine, close work with one. If your own experience has proven that you are adept with an electric shaver, by all means use it. But make sure it is clean and sharp. And proceed very, very slowly and carefully.

By far the best results can be achieved with an old-fashioned straight razor. An involuntary and sudden tracheotomy can also be achieved with a straight razor. Shaver, know thyself.

THE MIRROR

You will be doing close work. It is important that you be able to pay careful attention to detail. A magnifying shaving mirror will be of great use to you, even if you should later on regress to a naked chin. Ideally, the shaving mirror should be mounted near the regular bathroom mirror, so that you can scrutinize small areas while studying the overall effect with a minimum of eye-shifting.

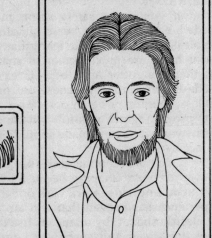

A CLEAR EYE AND A STEADY HAND

Do not attempt to begin pogonotrophy when you are tired. If you have a drink or two to bolster your courage, take your bolstered courage and go to bed, but stay away from the razor. It is essential that you approach the project calmly, coolly, and with all your faculties in perfect working order, because a slip at this time can be disastrous. Later, when your beard has grown in, an occasional minor mishap is of little consequence. But at this time, accuracy and precision are crucial.

For this very same reason, I advise you to lock yourself in the bathroom—alone—when you embark on beard-shaping. Women and children enjoy watching men shave, and no wonder: it is a ritual completely alien to them. Men, on the other hand, enjoy being watched. It seems to have a highly satisfying effect on the masculine ego. But I warn you: this is no time to give in to *machismo*. One titter, one snicker, one ill-timed wisecrack, and the whole project is literally down the drain. Even the best-intentioned female cannot resist offering a suggestion here and there, and this is bound to throw you off your course. (If I am to be accused of male chauvinism, so be it. I know what I know.)

Preparation

Even if you should decide, through some perversity, not to grow a beard after all, you will find this section very useful. I am about to describe the most efficient way to prepare a face for shaving. Attend.

Wash your face thoroughly with soap and warm water. The temperature of the water should be as hot as you can stand it, because hot water is the most efficient stubble-softener ever invented, as you will have discovered if you are clever enough to shave *after* your shower, instead of before. Work the soapy lather well into your beard, rubbing vigorously against the grain. Let the lather remain on your face for about a minute; then rinse it off, again with hot water, making sure to remove all the lather. Leave your face wet.

You are now ready to begin shaving. Soak the razor in hot water, the hotter the better. The edge of the blade which touches your face is so microscopically narrow that you will not feel the heat which the water has transmitted to the metal, but the scruffy little hairs on your face will, and shaving will be considerably more comfortable. Rinse the razor frequently, always in hot water.

It has probably not escaped your notice that I have so far failed to mention shaving cream. I never use it, and you probably will not need it if you follow the steps described above. If you feel an absolute necessity to use *something*, lather up again with the very same soap with which you washed; it will do nicely. But it is better to do without lather of any kind, especially if you are growing a beard, because the lather obscures outlines and borders. State Pharmacal Co., of Union, New Jersey, distributes a product called Amazing, a silicone substance which coats the edge of the blade and produces the same effect when shaving as lathering the face. It is not an easy product to find, but it is a boon to wearers of trimmed beards.

Outlining
Preparatory to your first shave as a bearded man, a few extra steps should be taken.

After you have washed your face thoroughly, dry it. Now, place the pictures from the vending machine on the mirror. Using them as a guide, draw the outline of the beard on your face with the eyebrow pencil. Take your time.

86

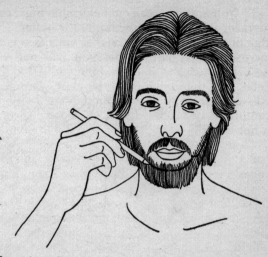

Remain calm. You are in the sanctity and seclusion of your own bathroom. If you make a mistake, take a facial tissue, rub off the eyebrow pencil, and begin again. Do not even think of picking up the razor until you are completely satisfied with the outline you have drawn.

Shaving

Now, wet your face again—very carefully so as not to smudge the outline. Pat the water on with your hand, and try to keep it outside the pencil line. Some water will no doubt dribble, but this is of no importance unless it obliterates a portion of the outline. If it does, merely dry the spot with a tissue and redraw the line.

Dip the razor into the water which, again, should be steaming hot, and shave. (An open window will keep the mirrors from clouding.)

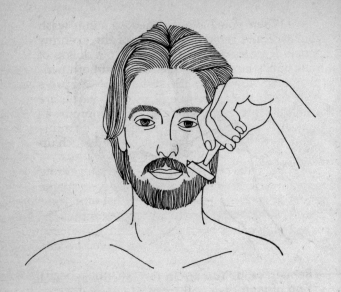

*Very important: Your razor strokes should begin
a fraction of an inch from the outline, not directly
on it.* Shave *away* from the outline, never toward
it. This may result in a less clean shave at first,
because of the grain pattern of your beard.
Never mind. You can always go back over the
difficult spots later. Again, proceed slowly and
carefully. Avoid using the long, sweeping
strokes to which you are accustomed, especially
when shaving near the outline. A better technique is to lay the blade against the skin and
then urge it forward with a series of very short,
careful strokes, each about a quarter- or a half-
inch in length. While shaving, pull the skin taut
with your fingers, being careful not to smudge
the pencil lines.

When you have finished shaving, wash your face and remove all traces of the eyebrow pencil. If necessary, help yourself to a dollop of your wife's face cream to remove stubborn pencil marks. Now study the result as it compares with the picture, bearing in mind that you are primarily interested in outline and contour, as opposed to density, which at best will be minimal. If necessary, take up the razor and touch up a bit.

You may, if you wish, use the eyebrow pencil to darken an occasional bare or sparse spot, but use it sparingly. Draw very short, light lines that resemble the hair, then blend them in by rubbing gently with your finger tip. Remember that such touch-ups should never be obvious.

Depending on the rate of your beard growth, you may find it necessary to be as careful during the next two or three shaves as you were on this first one. After that, you can relax a bit, because the hair will be dense enough to offer a slight resistance to the razor, providing a built-in signal to stop.

Congratulations. You are now a member of the bearded fraternity. *Now* go and have that drink. You deserve it.

7. THE GESTATION PERIOD

Despite the prevalent view that we live in a democratic society, many of us are often subjected to abuses which can best be described as minor intolerances. These intolerances are frequently expressed in the form of alleged humor, and if we fail to respond amiably, we are immediately accused of not being "good sports," which, as everyone knows, is un-American. Nevertheless, I am firmly convinced that so-called bad sportsmanship is the only thing which will save what shred of dignity we may have left.

Few people are so abused by these minor intolerances as are burgeoning pogonotrophers. You must remain firm and steadfast. You must refuse to smile when people call you Fuzzy Face. You must not join in japes or jests about the condition of your chin. I am not suggesting that you become abusive or belligerent. Rather, learn to assume an attitude of offended hauteur blended with quiet dignity. To do so is to cultivate a trait which will serve you well in a variety of circumstances. To fail to do so will most assuredly result in the consignment of your beard to the drainpipe and to the dark recesses of your unfulfilled fantasy world.

Paradoxically, you may prove to be your own worst enemy. You will almost certainly feel uncomfortable at a business conference or a social function with a three- or four-day growth on your chin. Furthermore, there will probably be some justification for your discomfort: a beard does not begin to look like a beard much before eight or 10 days, and really requires about three weeks before it becomes substantial. (I am talking about the average man. Some men can grow a full beard in less than a week, while one unfortunate friend of mine, after a year of diligent nonshaving, still looks as though his upper lip were dirty.)

The proper self-treatment during this period is both mental and physical in nature. Mentally, you must keep reminding yourself that it is only a matter of time before your beard will grow in—a handsome and complementary (as well as complimentary) testimony to your manhood. You should retain, indelibly impressed upon your mind's eye, the photograph of your face with the beard drawn on it. Soon, you will look like that picture. It will be well worth the wait.

Physically, the approach to the problem is twofold. First, if you can begin the period of nonshaving during your vacation or over a long weekend, you will already have the beginnings of a beard when you return to the job. Second, when you finally do have to face the public, wear your best clothes and avoid informality of dress. A new suit, crisp shirt, modish tie, and spit-polished shoes can hardly be interpreted, even by the most insensitive clod, as the garb of a bum, despite the unshaven chin. While I do not normally encourage ostentation, this might be a good time to wear one or two pieces of expensive jewelry—if you own any, that is, and happen to live in a low-crime area, such as the Mojave Desert.

Above all, remember that other people's attitudes will be directly influenced and determined by yours. If you are self-deprecating and apologetic, your best friends and closest relatives will descend upon you like a school of piranha. If, on the other hand, you discuss your beard, sparse as it may yet be, with dignity, aplomb, and just a soupçon of aloofness, you will gain the respect and admiration of all but the most boorish, whose company you should probably avoid in any case.

A Beard of a Different Color

You may be surprised to discover that your beard is a different color from the hair on your head. Do not be alarmed. This is perfectly normal and, as a matter of fact, provides an added element of interest. My hair (what is left of it) is brown, but my beard is predominantly black, dotted with an occasional red-brown highlight and gray striations. When conversation lags, I can always rely on my beard to provide the basis for a discussion on The Vagaries of Nature, a topic which can lead almost anywhere.

From time to time, but especially in the early stages, your beard will itch. There is only one rational way to cope with this problem: scratch it. (The alternative—ignoring it—requires a special kind of masochism.) *How* you scratch it depends entirely upon your personality and propensity. There are three common scratching techniques.

SURREPTITIOUS

This method involves scratching the beard while pretending to do something else. It can be done in a variety of ways. A rather histrionic method is to drop something on the floor and then, while picking it up, hastily scrape the fingernails over the offending spot while no one can see you. A variation is to call people's attention to something else in the room and scratch when they turn away to look.

The easiest way to scratch surreptitiously is to pretend to do something else in the area of the face, such as blowing or rubbing your nose, adjusting your glasses, straightening your necktie, etc. While the *apparent* activity is going on, one or two fingers deftly attend to the real problem.

PENSIVE

This method is really semisurreptitious. Develop the habit of rubbing or stroking your chin when thinking something over, in the manner of a physician who pretends to be mulling over a patient's symptoms, while he is actually wondering how he can get away long

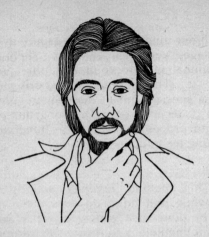

enough to call someone to find out what is wrong. An occasional "Hmmm" lends considerable credence to this technique. When you have an itch, hold out for a few seconds—just long enough for someone to give you an opportunity to say "Hmmm" and thoughtfully rub your chin.

OPEN

Frankly, I prefer this technique. When I itch, I scratch, and I do not care who knows or sees. Admittedly, one must exercise a modicum of discretion with respect to certain parts of the body, but not when it comes to the beard. As in all things, dignity and decorum must prevail. There is nothing wrong with open scratching as long as it is done quietly and unobtrusively. One should not claw at one's skin as though a swarm of fleas had just established residence. At least, not in company.

94

Coping with Objections

There is always the possibility that even in this permissive age, you will meet open and serious resistance to the idea of your growing a beard. Such resistance may come from your wife (girlfriend, mother, landlady, maiden aunt, etc.; see Chapter 5), your employer, customers and clients, friends, children — in fact, from virtually anyone with whom you have frequent contact. As previously stated, these people can make your life miserable and ultimately compel you to divest yourself of your beard, adding considerably to your store of frustration and nonfulfillment. If your pogonotrophy is to succeed, these resisters must be dealt with. As you may have guessed by now, there are several ways of doing so.

SELF-ASSERTIVENESS

You are your own man; no one should be able to tell you what to do or when to do it, as long as you are not interfering with anyone else's well-being. As a free, independent, mature citizen in good standing, there is not a reason in the world why you should not grow a beard if you wish to do so. Be strong. Be firm. Be determined. Remain steadfast. Good luck.

FAIR PLAY

She: "I think your beard looks lousy." You: "Of course it looks lousy. I've only had it three days. Even a baby looks lousy after only three days. Tell you what. Let's give it around six weeks, so that it has a chance to grow in. After that, if you still think it looks lousy, I'll

shave it off." She: "Promise?" You: "Promise."
She: "Well, okay; but remember, if I don't like
it after six weeks, off it comes!" You: *Silence,
followed by an indulgent smile and a kiss on the
cheek.*

If you promise not to blab this all over
town, I will let you in on a secret: the Fair Play,
or Wait-Six-Weeks Approach, is pure, un-
adulterated flummery. Your beard will probably
be as good as it will ever get after three or four
weeks. But it will take a full six weeks for her to
get used to it. If she holds you to your promise
at the end of the "trial" period, then you may
reasonably assume that she will never fully accept it. How you proceed after that depends entirely on your relationship with her.

Above all, *leave it to her to remember the
deadline.* Never, never say: "Well, kiddo, the six
weeks are up. Still think I ought to shave off the
beard?" He who seeks trouble will surely find it.
Simply allow the six weeks to glide by, unno-
ticed by you and, hopefully, by her. In most
cases, you will encounter no further difficulty.
Do not be surprised if you overhear her saying
to someone at a party: "Well, I was against it at
first, but now I rather like it." How much she
likes it also depends on you. (See Chapter 9.)

THE POOR-ME APPROACH
Some men have mastered the art of play-
ing on other people's sympathies. They get what
they want by whining, cajoling, and pretending
that they feel unloved and unwanted. (I under-
stand that some successful seductions have been
worked this way. I cannot imagine how.) Ulti-

mately, the petitionee relents, if only to stem the sickening flow of self-pity issuing from the petitioner. Such acquiescence is usually accompanied by contempt, which is richly deserved.

THE BUILDUP

People who lead ordinary, uncomplicated, conservative lives are frequently unable to cope with dramatic changes. In such cases, it is not the beard *per se* which upsets them; it is the (relatively) sudden and radical change in your appearance. These people need to be gently guided. Begin by lengthening your sideburns somewhat. When they have gotten used to that, add a mustache, followed by an Underlip or a Vandyke, and then on to whatever style you want to remain with. This is an extremely effective, if tedious, method which requires a great deal of patience.

The particular technique you use may vary with the individual and the circumstances. For example, a salesman who has topped his quota every month for the past year, and who is married to a woman the mere sight of whom sends the pulse racing, may find it best to be self-assertive with his employer, while using the Fair Play or Poor-Me method at home. Feel free to adapt any of the methods, or combinations thereof, to your own personal needs.

Children

Because of their as yet incompletely developed intellects, many children are frightened by bearded men. Do not let this factor deter you. An occasional trauma is good for a child, as it

97

trains him for the vicissitudes of life which he must ultimately face. It is also good for you. Other people's children will leave you alone, even to the point of avoiding being in the same room with you when you come to visit. Your own experience has probably proven by now that this is greatly to be desired. As for your own children, if you ever expect to have an even chance of defending yourself against them, you could do worse than to have them begin life by being a little terrified of you.

On occasion, you may encounter a little girl who will like your beard and will ask for permission to touch it. She will coo, gurgle, and smile. Such a child bears watching; if the age difference is not too great, her friendship may be worth cultivating as she emerges from puberty. One three-year-old siren recently described my face as "fluffy." It will be interesting to observe her development.

8. CARE AND FEEDING OF THE BEARD

Just as a well-groomed beard is a handsome addition to a man's appearance, an ill-kept one will damage his image, regardless of what he does to the rest of his person. It is essential, therefore, that the beard be given meticulous care, with special attention to cleanliness.

Washing

Your beard should be washed whenever you bathe or shower, more frequently if you are a careless eater. Ordinary soap and water will usually suffice. If you have some special problem, such as dandruff or extremely dry hair, you will have to do more, but basic washing is essential.

Use a good, rich lather and work it very thoroughly into the beard, rubbing vigorously. Rinse well, making sure to remove all the soap. Any residue will become thick and gummy, causing the hair to mat.

If you have a very full beard and connected sideburns, you may find it convenient to wash all the hair on your head at the same time. There is no harm in using shampoo on your beard. In fact, as you shall soon learn, it may do some good.

Incidentally, extensive beard-trimming is best done just before showering. Beard hairs which fall on your body are then easily washed off and run down the drain.

Combing and Brushing

Use a thin, long, flat comb such as is used by your barber, to work out the tangles and smooth out your beard. Follow with a vigorous brushing.

The best kind of brush is one which is fairly thin and has very stiff bristles. You may have to do some hunting about for a suitable one, but with diligence you should be able to locate a brush which meets your requirements. Again, I caution you to avoid being conned into purchasing an expensive brush unless doing so appeals to some pride of ownership in you. It makes no difference whether you use a beard brush with bristles made from unborn Patagonian hedgehog or one whose bristles are extruded plastic (which, incidentally, is what I use), as long as the bristles are stiff, firm, and wiry.

Brush your beard in the direction in which you want the hairs to lie. Generally, a continual downward motion will suffice, with some rounding off along the jawline and under the chin for short beards.

Always dry your beard before combing and brushing.

Trimming

There are several tools which are very useful in pogonoculture:

A pair of long, thin barber's shears.

A pair of very short scissors with rounded points.

A long, thin, flat comb (as described above).

A home hair trimmer.

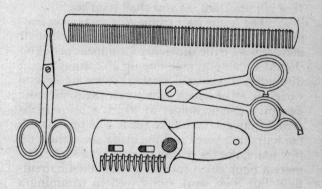

The barber's shears afford excellent control when snipping and trimming. Their length and thinness make it possible to reach almost any part of the face without obstructing your view or compelling you to go through joint-dislocating contortions.

The short, round-nosed scissors, which can be obtained in a store which sells cutlery or in any shop with a good stock of manicure implements, are used for clipping unsightly tufts of hair growing from the ears and the nose. The rounded points aid in preventing an inadvertent punctured eardrum or an extra nostril. Hair should never be plucked from the ears and nose. This is not only quite painful but also invites infection.

The barber-type comb, because of its shape, offers the same advantages as the shears, with the added characteristic of being somewhat flatter than most ordinary household combs. This is important, as you shall soon see.

The home hair trimmer is extremely useful for thinning out sideburns and beards. (It may prove a trifle unwieldy for mustaches.) You should be able to pick one up at a drugstore or through a direct-mail catalog. There are several varieties, all of which incorporate the same basic design: a plastic holder in which a blade is inserted between comblike teeth. The teeth comb the hairs into place and the blade slices them off (the hairs, not the teeth). I have found such trimmers a poor substitute for professional haircutting, but they work quite well in trimming a beard. I recommend that you stay with the kind of trimmer which uses ordinary razor blades, because those equipped with special blades may pose something of a problem when the time comes to replace them.

When using the trimmer, be certain that the blade is first immersed in very hot water. This will enable you to work on hair as dry as hay. If, however, the trimmer blade is dry, your bellows of pain will be heard in the next county. Hold the trimmer at about a 45° angle. The more horizontal it is, the less cutting it will do. The more vertical it is, the more likely you are to strip off more hair than you intended. As with any razor blade, go slowly, be careful, and use short strokes. The trimmer is a stopgap, for interim care and for touching up. Your best work will be accomplished with the comb and shears.

Never use unguarded shears on your beard. Run the comb through the portion you want to trim, hold the comb in place, and snip off the hairs that protrude through the comb.

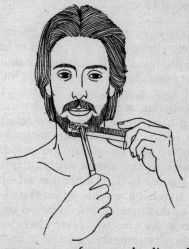

This will assure you of an evenly clipped beard, as no hair will be shorter or longer than the thickness of the comb. If the comb is too thin for your preference, angle it until it exposes the desired length of hair. If the comb is too thick (a highly unlikely contingency), use it anyway and then go over the beard with the hair trimmer. The trimmer can also be used for hard-to-reach places.

If you prefer to use an electric shaver, follow the same basic principle. Run the shaver head over the comb so that you do not cut too closely.

It is, of course, possible to trim a beard with an ordinary razor. By using a sharp blade, a hot razor, and light, skimming action, you will find that the hairs can be trimmed quite easily this way. You will also find the next section of vital interest to you.

Gouges, Holes, and Bald Spots

Overenthusiasm or impatience frequently result in the removal of more hair than originally intended, usually in one clump. One can invariably spot a pogonotropher who trims his beard with an ordinary razor, because somewhere in his whiskers there is a small clearing through which a patch of skin virtually gleams. This mishap also occurs to overconfident types who resort to the shears without troubling to employ the comb. (I am embarrassed—but nonetheless driven by a sense of honesty—to admit that all of this information is based on personal experience. As a matter of fact, I believe this may have been the underlying cause of the pogonotomy mentioned in the Introduction.)

Some men have facial bald spots on which the hair will not grow or grows very sparsely, giving the effect of a ragged, mottled beard. For

can prove to be traumatic; but you will be saved
by the realization that, sooner or later, your
beard will grow back again.

Some men have a summer beard and a
winter beard. As the cold climate sets in, they
allow their beards to grow in more fully, pro-

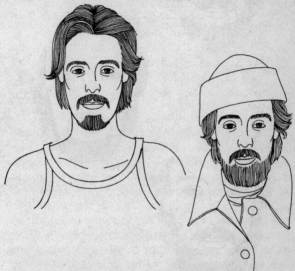

viding for themselves a cozy insulation against
wintry blasts. As the seasons change, they snip
away more and more, so that by the time the
roses are in bloom, the beard is reduced to a
closely cropped, small Vandyke.

Others keep changing the shape of the
beard while retaining the overall size. Thus,
one month they will have a pointed beard, the
next month a rounded one, then a squared-off
one. Detaching a mustache for a few weeks and

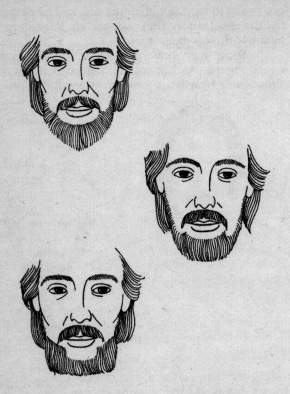

then letting it grow back to meet the beard once more is a pleasant, diverting exercise in aesthetics.

Try combing the beard in different ways. The very same quantity of hair can look quite different combed straight down, rounded under the chin, or parted in the middle and swept outward.

Again, the shape of the beard can be retained, while variations can be tried with regard to how far back the beard goes. It can end just behind the chin, extend clear back to the Adam's apple, or terminate anywhere in between.

Fool around. You have nothing to lose but your beard, and that loss is only temporary.

The Beard as a Symbol of Strength

During the Dark Ages (*ca.* 1964 A.D.), I was advised by several employment agency types to shave my beard in order to facilitate jobhunting. I steadfastly refused to do so. I am, by nature and by design, a beard wearer. My chin might be naked, but my psyche would still be bearded and a prospective employer had the right, I felt, to know that I have the personality of a beard wearer, a pogonophile, a pogonotropher. Whether such an employer would find that an asset or a liability would depend, of course, on his particular outlook, but whatever that might be, I would not deceive him. Thus is character built.

If we have emerged somewhat from the Dark Ages, we can hardly claim to have entered the Age of Enlightenment. Pogonotrophers are still subjected to boorish deprecation on all sides. Such prejudice must be recognized for what it is and dealt with politely but firmly. Thus is character strengthened.

A man's only reason for growing a beard should be that he wants to do so. A man should never joke about, make excuses for, or apologize for his beard, for thus is character weakened.

123

The Beard as a Life-Style

Throughout this work, I have constantly admonished you to go slowly, to proceed with care, to approach every situation concerning your beard calmly, easily, contemplatively, unhurriedly. If you heed my advice, you will find that your entire life is vastly improved. Consider:

At meals, in order to avoid unsightly spills on your beard, you will eat slowly and carefully. Each morsel will be lifted to your lips with caution, and, while you are preserving the cleanliness of your beard, you are also heightening the anticipation of the taste of the food. Your wine will be sipped with equal care, to keep it from spilling into your beard; but at the same time it will flow gently over your taste buds, permeating your mouth with its savor, instead of merely sloshing down your gullet like so much slop. Protecting your beard may be your primary purpose, but the ultimate reward is the full appreciation of good food and drink which can only be achieved by an unhurried approach.

After dinner, you will light your tobacco with caution, cognizant of the fact that a beard aflame is embarrassing at best and dangerous at worst. You will smoke more diligently for the purpose of keeping embers and ashes out of your beard. But in the process you will enjoy the flavor of the tobacco more. Cigarette smokers who grow beards have been known to switch to cigars and pipes, or to the more flavorful, aromatic foreign cigarettes.

In the love chamber, you will know that a roughly managed beard can scratch, irritate,

124

or tickle, while a well-handled one can excite and titillate. So you will move very slowly, lingering over each hollow and rise, inhaling the precious perfumes, fully appreciating the vast territory of the human female form in all its evocative nuances, reaping rewards often unknown to beardless men.

And so it goes: Once you have discovered the pleasure and usefulness of an unhurried, unharried approach to life's situations, you will find yourself employing the technique in everything you do. You will think before you speak. You will listen to both sides of a question before making a decision. You will not allow others to pressure you into rash moves.

Is it not possible, you may well ask, to achieve all this *without* growing a beard? The answer is yes, but that is the subject of another book. Written, I suppose, by a psychiatrist— with a beard, no doubt.

I leave you with the words of William Shakespeare, the bearded bard who said almost everything worth saying, and said it better than anyone else:

> *Jove, in his next commodity of hair,*
> *send thee a beard!*

such people there is no help. The solutions for holes and gouges will in some cases work for bald spots, but they are at best stopgaps, as it were. The man afflicted with bald spots should endeavor to evolve a beard style which works around, rather than incorporates, those spots. If this cannot be done, he might do well to abandon the idea of a beard altogether. There is something unpleasantly leprous-looking about a patchy beard.

Handling bald spots on the chin is not unlike handling them on the head. In both locations, it comes down to a matter of how wide an area the spot covers and how abundant the adjacent hair is. Thus, a bare spot in a beard can often be covered over by allowing the surrounding hair to grow a bit longer, and training it to grow over the naked skin. If you have not returned the eyebrow pencil to its rightful owner, use it to touch up and fill in a bit.

Trimming the Mustache

At the risk of being accused of condescension, permit me to remind you that when you trim your mustache, *make sure your mouth is closed,* unless you enjoy spending an hour picking tiny hairs off your tongue.

If you have chosen a mustache style which requires that the ends stand away from the face (e.g., the RAF or Handlebar), you should begin to direct its growth from the very outset. When you first shape the mustache, determine the line at which the mustache is to stand alone. This will constitute the outer boundary when you shave. As your mustache thickens, comb

105

the hairs straight down over your upper lip and shave carefully along those predetermined boundary lines. Now comb the mustache horizontally, outward from the center toward both ends. You will soon find that the ends have

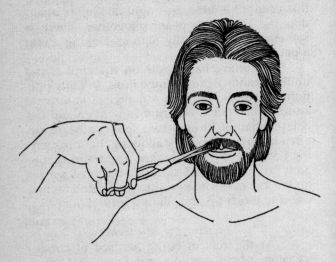

reached the desired length. Continue shaving in this manner, using your barber's shears to snip off excess length and to keep the ends even.

On the other hand, if you prefer a flat, straight mustache, use the comb-and-shears technique described above. You may find it easier to comb up, toward the nose. In addition, comb the mustache straight down and snip off the hairs which extend below the line where the upper lip begins. If you forget to keep your mouth closed once, you will never forget again.

Standaway mustache styles may prove difficult to control at first. If you can find a store which sells mustache wax, it will help immeasurably. To the best of my knowledge, there is only one brand on the market. It is manufactured by Ed. Pinaud and is called *Pomade Hongroise*. (This means "Hungarian pomade"; the approximate pronunciation is *poe-MAD hong-rWAZ.) Pomade Hongroise* comes in very small tubes and is available in five colors, ranging from black to silver-gray. When rubbed into the mustache, it darkens the hair slightly and gives it a not unattractive sheen. A very little goes a long, long way. A dedicated pharmacist or barber should be able to obtain a tube for you, and that one tube ought to last you so long that by the time you are ready for a second, you will be ordering the silver-gray.

In the absence of said dedicated merchants, purchase a little pure beeswax from your druggist. It liquefies when rubbed between the fingers and is virtually odorless and colorless.

Pomade Hongroise and beeswax are of a rather heavy consistency and are therefore impractical for beards and sideburns. A light hairdressing, such as the clear, water-soluble hair creams (Score, Groom & Clean, etc.) or a liquid, will help keep stray hairs in place on cheek and chin.

Economy is the watchword when using any of these cosmetics on the beard. Even the most highly advertised "nongreasy" hair preparation will make a beard look oily and matted. The best way to determine how much is enough

107

is to dispense what you estimate to be the proper amount—then use half of it. You can always add a little more if necessary, but if you apply too much at the outset, you will have the devil's own time trying to remove the excess. In any case, as soon as your beard and mustache show signs of behaving themselves, discard the dressing unless you have unusually dry facial hair. Such preparations should be used to train and control your beard, not glue it into place.

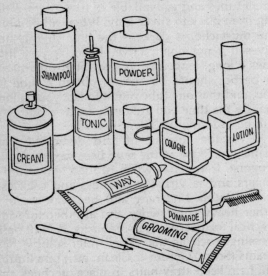

After-shave lotions and colognes should never be rubbed into the beard. Most if not all of these preparations have a high alcohol content, and alcohol is anathema to natural hair oils. A dab or so about the ears, around the neck, and around the wrists (so the lady can tell how sexy you smell when you light her cigarette) will stand you in good stead.

Some men discover, upon rubbing or scratching their beards, a gentle blizzard descending on their chests. It is somewhat disturbing. Having taken the precautions prescribed by Madison Avenue to spray everywhere from crotch to armpits, having gargled with pesticide to avoid breathy offense, and having lacerated one's scalp with the latest version of foaming kerosene to destroy all life which may have found its way into one's silken locks—having undergone all these tortures, it is disconcerting indeed to discover that one's beard is infected with dandruff. Disconcerting, yes. Incurable? No. In all likelihood, if you have "beardruff" (a word I invented for convenience's sake), you probably also have dandruff and have by now discovered a shampoo or some other product which controls it. That product will also control beardruff in most cases. When you wash your hair, wash your beard with the same shampoo. What works on your scalp should work on your chin. If it does not, you have three alternatives: (1) Experiment with various products until you find one which works. This may mean using one nostrum for your scalp and another for your chin. (2) Consult a dermatologist. (3) Ignore it. Try not to scratch your beard in public; when you do scratch, lightly—and as unobtrusively as possible—brush the flakes off your lapels and necktie. There is, of course, a fourth choice: shave off your beard. That, however, is not a solution; it is a cop-out.

Cleaning Up

Now that you have washed, combed, clipped, trimmed, and dressed your beard, take the few minutes necessary to clean up. Wash all the implements thoroughly and dry those that are likely to rust or mildew. Remove all razor blades, or at least loosen the razor and hair trimmer sufficiently to allow drying air to circulate through them.

And for God's sake, clean the sink! Your wife will never give you a moment's peace, no matter how much she likes your beard, if you leave her with a wash basin that looks as though the Hound of the Baskervilles had slept in it. Lest the suggestion that you do even this minimal amount of housework offend your *machismo*, I hasten to explain that cleaning up after a beard-trim is simplicity itself. A moistened wad of tissue, either facial or toilet, works wonders. A few deft swipes will clean away even the tiniest of hairs, which for some reason have an affinity for wet tissue.

Professional Care

If you have the misfortune to be a congenital *klutz*, disregard all of the foregoing. Go back to the part in Chapter 5 where you have drawn a beard on your photograph. Take the photograph to your barber and show him what you want done.

Even if you manage fairly well in the shaping, cultivation, and maintenance of your beard, a visit to the local tonsorium will do you no harm. With every third haircut or so, ask the barber to prune your beard. *Do not entrust your*

110

beard to an unknown barber. I have yet to find the barber who will not botch the job when working on the beard of someone who is not a regular customer. If someone recommends a barber to you, use that person's name when you sit down in the chair. If necessary, invent a name. "Melvin Weltschmerz told me you're the best barber in town. I hope he's right." The barber is not likely to know the name of every one of his customers. He may spend the next month asking some of his regulars: "Are you Melvin Weltschmerz?" Never mind. That's his problem. Your problem is getting a decent haircut and a proper beard-trim. It is a question of self-defense.

A good barber is worth his weight in gold. Tip him well. He deserves it. And you deserve the kind of treatment a good tip guarantees.

With your beard properly groomed, you are ready for action. Let us now discuss the action.

9. THE SENSUOUS BEARD

"During the past two years I have had to spend periods of several weeks on a remote island in comparative isolation. In these conditions I noticed that my beard growth diminished, but the day before I was due to leave the island it increased again, to reach unusually high rates during the first day or two on the mainland. Intrigued by these initial observations, I have carried out a more detailed study and have come to the conclusion that the stimulus for increased beard growth is related to the resumption of sexual activity."

This forthright pronouncement is the opening paragraph of an article entitled "Effects of Sexual Activity on Beard Growth in Man," published in the May 30, 1970, issue of *Nature*, a highly reputable—if somewhat dry—British scientific journal. The author, a capable young scientist whose anonymity was preserved by the magazine, kept careful records, weighing the hairs which he collected in his electric shaver. The article is accompanied by graphs and charts to demonstrate that, as the weekend with its promise of female companionship approached, there was a marked acceleration in beard growth, increasing as much as 20% by Friday. *"Even the presence of particular female company in the absence of intercourse, after a period of separation, usually caused an obvious increase in beard growth . . . it seems that beard growth in man is a much-neglected parameter of hormone activity that can readily be quantified."*

In simple English, anticipation starts the juices flowing, and those juices fertilize the beard. (That is not all they fertilize, if one is not careful.) Thus, we now have scientific evidence of the correlation between beards and sexiness. This is not to suggest that the reader engage in a program of abstinence/anticipation in order to stimulate a recalcitrant beard, but rather to point up the importance of beards to sexual activity, and vice versa.

Your Beard and Your Woman

There is a profound wisdom in women which is so universal that it is impossible for a mere layman to determine whether it is instinctual, intuitive, or culturally instilled. It is there, nevertheless, and men who do not resemble matinee idols should be grateful for its existence, for it enables a woman to judge and evaluate a man by more than the mere superficialities of physical appearance. Whatever your basic character, personality, faults, assets, vices, and virtues may be, they are not likely to change because you have grown a beard. Your woman knows this, and if she insists that you are "not

113

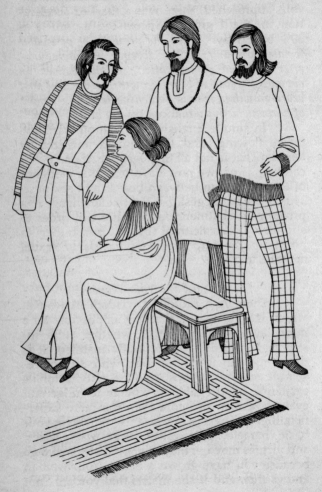

114

the type" to wear a beard it is because she has certain associations to beards which her wisdom tells her are wrong for you. You may disagree with her at first, perhaps to the point where you go your separate ways; but do not be surprised if, in the long run, she proves to be right.

Chances are, however, that she will accept your beard; and if she is less than enthusiastic about it, she will at least tolerate it. Under such circumstances, your beard must never become a source of hardship and discomfort to her. Read the section, further on in this chapter, on "Bearded Lovemaking." You owe it to her.

The Beard on the Prowl

Feminine wisdom notwithstanding, women do have certain likes and dislikes. A bearded, footloose bachelor must be aware, early on, that some women simply do not like beards, just as some women do not like red hair, eyeglasses, French accents, woolen neckties, etc. A mature man knows that he cannot have everything, and therefore concentrates on obtaining the best of what he *can* have.

There are, of course, a great many women who *do* like beards. In my own experience, these invariably prove to be women who are intelligent and literate. They are good conversationalists, are endowed with a keen sense of humor, and have a flair for adventure and experimentation while eschewing recklessness for its own sake. Such women have apparently found bearded men highly satisfying and fulfilling in a variety of ways.

Your beard will make social contact considerably easier, because at parties and other occasions, beard-loving women tend to gravitate, almost without realizing it, toward the hirsute faces in the room. But it is not the beard *per se* which attracts them. It is what the beard promises: intelligence, wit, individuality, manliness. A woman can penetrate a pretentious façade like a hot knife going through butter, and if a beard advertises merchandise which the supplier is unable to deliver, its wearer will never do business in that marketplace. Better to be unbearded and honest than to be hairy-chinned and disreputable.

Bearded Lovemaking

It is interesting to note that none of the sex manuals includes a section on the employment and/or deployment of the beard in the act of love. Perhaps their single-initialled ("J," "M") or multiple-degreed (M.D., Ph.D., Sc.D.) authors believe the number of bearded lovers to be too small to be concerned about. I prefer to think that they assume that a bearded man has advanced beyond the need of sex manuals. The fact remains, however, that the beard does introduce a new and different element into the art of love, which requires some study and attention.

Bearded lovemaking can be simplicity itself if you remember two rules which are so self-evident that they are easily overlooked: (1) *A woman's skin is much more sensitive than a man's.* (2) *Wherever your face goes, your beard goes with it.* The combination of these two factors will, without exception, evoke at least one of three reactions, from a woman: (1) You will tickle her. (2) You will scratch or irritate her skin. (3) You will cause an odd sensation which she has never before experienced and which she will either (a) hate or (b) love. There will be variations, combinations, and contradictions (*e.g.*, scratching in one place, tickling in another, tickling a place on one occasion, scratching that same place on another occasion, etc.), but there will always be *something*.

If you are exploring new—if not necessarily virgin—territory, you must proceed with great caution. Few things can turn a woman off faster than the sensation that a delicate and intimate part of her body is being scoured with Brillo. Equally devastating is an attack of the giggles brought on by indiscriminate tickling. As for that third, odd sensation mentioned above, her reaction will be indicated by a comment such as: "Oh, I've never felt anything quite like *that* before!" How you proceed from there depends on whether the comment is followed by a long, quavery sigh or a terse "Yech!"

I will be the first to concede that, in the heat of passion, it is usually difficult to keep memorized axioms in the forefront of one's consciousness—even such simple ones as the two mentioned earlier. But if you qualify as any kind of lover at all, you should at least be responsive to signals. As your beard wanders hither and yon, take heed of sighs, winces, coos, whimpers, groans, gurgles, moans, etc. If you are unable to determine if and when such signs indicate pleasure or pain, stop wasting your time reading this book and go out to get some sorely needed practice; your education is deficient in areas much more important than pogonotrophy.

Kissing

One of the most important reasons for keeping a beard and mustache well trimmed is that it keeps hair away from the lips. No woman, no matter how much she likes beards, enjoys having a mouthful of hair bestowed upon her. As a matter of fact, she may not even like the feel of your beard against her face. This can frequently be overcome by proceeding gradually. Begin with an almost full pucker, creating a sort

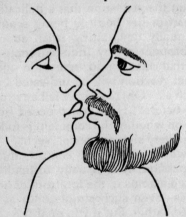

of lippy barrier between her face and your whiskers. The pucker can be diminished gradually as the situation progresses. In this way, she will not only become used to the feel of your beard but, hopefully, will be so distracted by the other things that are happening that she will hardly notice.

To sum up: Chances are that if the lady likes the beard on your face, she will not object, and in fact may enjoy, having it on some part of *her*. Never force the issue. With care, consideration, and easy, unhurried experimentation, you may discover that your beard has sexual properties and applications which are limited only by your inhibitions and your imagination. If you can manage to repress the one, I have no doubt that the lady will help you to express the other.

10. THE ART OF WEARING A BEARD

I wish I could tell you that you now know all there is to know about wearing a beard. Alas, I cannot, for there are some things no one can teach you, things which you must learn for yourself. The best I can do is to supply a few general guidelines which I hope will direct you along certain paths — paths which you must, ultimately, tread alone, until you find your way. If you cannot find a path, or do not approve of the ones you do find, do not hesitate to make your own, for beard wearers through the centuries have been pathfinders and trailblazers.

The Beard as a Hobby

Your beard is your very own; feel free to do with it as you wish. Never be afraid to experiment. The worst that can happen is that you make a mistake and will have to start over from the very beginning. If you become as attached to your beard as I have become to mine, that